Wykes:

MORNING
EEPING
ND

RVEY OF AMERICAN LITERATURE

abazon of Tara: THE BRABAZON STORY
unter: HUNTER'S TRACKS
Wilfred H. Scott-Shawe: MARINER'S TALE
ayner: THE GREAT YACHT RACE

ND HIS ENEMY

E THAMES

efinitive study

a history of civil and military transatlantic

ENINGRAD
MPSHIRE REGIMENT

SELVES: comic drawings about women

F AMATEUR DRAMATICS

DOCT

Alan Wykes

DOCTOR CARDANO

Physician Extraordinary

FREDERICK MULLER

*First published in Great Britain 1969
by Frederick Muller Ltd., Fleet Street, London, E.C.4*

Copyright © 1969 by Alan Wykes

*Printed and bound in Great Britain by
The Garden City Press Limited
Letchworth, Hertfordshire*

SBN: 584 10063 9

To
ALEC BAYNES

Acknowledgements

Medieval Latin and Renaissance Italian are not my strong points. The late T. H. White helped me with the first and Professor Daria Tiranti with the latter. The specialized languages of medicine, pharmacology, and mathematics also needed a great deal of unravelling for me. Much of it was done by Frank Allen of the Forest Group Hospital Management Committee, Dr T. Anwyl-Davies, Professor Francis Camps, Edgar Schlesinger, Dr Victor Goldman, and Dr C. H. Talbot of the Wellcome Institute of the History of Medicine. Dr Alec Baynes gave me a considered modern opinion of Cardano's diagnosis, prognosis, and treatment of Archbishop Hamilton's illness. Robert Fabian gave me the clue that led me to the transcript of the trial of Giovanni Cardano—perhaps not surprisingly, since he has been for most of his life a detective. Gastone Silvano of the Institute of Italian Affairs and the several information officers and librarians of the Italian Embassy in London were always helpful, while the staffs of the British Museum Library, the London Library, the Bibliothèque Nationale, and the Biblioteca Nazionale Centrale were as indefatigable as ever in producing books, photostats, and answers to questions. My thanks to them all.

A.W.

Illustrations

*The illustration facing page 149 is from the British Museum;
the others from Radio Times Hulton Picture Library*

Introduction

I first encountered the name of Gerolamo Cardano—Jerome Cardan in English, Hieronymus Cardanus in Latin—when I was writing a book on gambling. Whichever name you call him by, it was he who first propounded the mathematical theory of probability, which has much to do with that subject. But in reading his *Book on Games of Chance* and Mr Oystein Ore's monograph *Cardano, the Gambling Scholar* I found that there was far more to Cardano than a headful of algebraic equations. He was also an inventor, an astrologer, an astronomer, a philosopher, and a doctor. On the side, as it were, he was skilled in divination by palmistry and geomancy; and he was the first to recognize that much could be told about human character by the study of physiognomy and handwriting. His own character combined intellectual brilliance, emotional instability, moral courage, and a pathetically misplaced devotion to his scoundrelly children. He achieved great fame in his lifetime but was brought to ruin and obscurity by his sons and the bitter enmity of another scholar, Nicolo Tartaglia. Today it is hard to find anyone who has ever heard of him, though his name is unwittingly mentioned by aficianados of the motor-car every time they refer to the cardan-shaft, a mechanical device he invented.

In medicine, Cardano ranks with Hippocrates, Galen, Maimonides, and other physicians of classical and medieval times. He fought against prejudice and the superstitions that in the dark ages had become associated with the study of physical ills. His brilliance as a diagnostician and his researches in tuberculosis, asthma, and the venereal diseases proved to be of immense value to later giants in the field of medicine.

He wrote more than two hundred books on everything that interested him, including himself, and many of them were bestsellers in his lifetime. As a fashionable doctor he was called to the service of kings, princes, and prelates; and by his cure of the asthmatical illness of the Archbishop of Scotland he changed the course of British history. Clearly, he was a man worth writing about; but in fact very little has been written about him in English. An impressive 600-page *Life* by Henry Morley was published in 1854, and what was virtually a rewritten and condensed version of that biography was turned out by W. G. Waters in 1898. Both these are afflicted with Victorian turgidity and would seem unapproachable by today's readers even if they were available. There are a few studies like Mr Ore's of particular aspects of his work, but nothing that sketches the man moving within the epoch of the Renaissance, Reformation, and counter-Reformation. This profile is meant to do that, no more; though it does reveal some aspects of Cardano's nature that were suppressed by Morley and Waters in the interests of Victorian pudency. He did not suppress them in his autobiographical works and I do not feel called upon to be a Victorian in an Elizabethan epoch.

Prologue

It is historically convenient to date the beginning of the Renaissance as 1414 and its end as 1527, though no arbitrary dates can really be pinned to the movement that was in effect the beginning of modern Europe. But on 1 November 1414 the council of cardinals convened by Pope John XXIII met at Lake Constance, their object being to try once again to bridge the schism that for more than thirty years had riven the church.* The climactic cause of the rift was the election to the papacy of Urban VI in 1378. Urban was an Italian (his name was Bartholomeus Prignanus) and he was put upon the throne, the college of cardinals said, because the citizens of Rome had threatened to riot if they were not given an Italian pope. The cardinals' real choice had been a Frenchman, Robertus de Gebennis, and within six months of electing Prignanus to save bloodshed they pronounced him deposed and de Gebennis reigning in his stead. Prignanus, however, declined to be deposed; and naturally he gained the support of Italy as well as of eastern Europe and England. Equally, de Gebennis was supported by the French emperor Charles V, by Scotland, and by the countries of the Iberian peninsula. The two rival popes and their successors reigned in bitter conflict, one in Rome and the other in Avignon, until 1414, when the council of Constance began the long meeting that was to end nearly four years later with the schism bridged, if somewhat tremulously, by the election of Oddone Colonna in 1417. Oddone was to reign as Pope

* The more familiar John XXIII was Cardinal Roncalli, who was elected in 1953. But he was in fact the twenty-fourth to assume the name of John. The modern chronology of popes excludes the anti-popes, of whom the convener of the Lake Constance conference was one.

Martin V—though not entirely undisputedly—until his death in
1431.

Looking back from the 20th century, in which the importance of the church has declined, it is difficult to grasp the effect
the division of papal authority had upon the daily life of the
christian world. No one can say with incontrovertible authority
when the see of Rome was founded or who was its first bishop.
But since the christian faith accepts the tradition of St Peter as
the founder of the church and of the apostolic succession it
clearly was of tremendous importance that the papal line should
be preserved unwaveringly. The absolute authority of Christ's
vicar on earth is no matter for disputed identity. So the schism
was not simply a question of whether christians accepted the
pontificates of a Roman or Avignonese line of popes: it was a
threat to the unity of christianity as a concept.

The simultaneous pontificates of Urban VI and Clement VII
(as Robertus de Gebennis chose to be called) were by no means
the first manifestation of the schism. There were popes and
anti-popes (as the more dubiously elected of the rivals for the
papacy are called) for centuries before the election of Urban
and Clement brought the papal succession into widespread,
open, and dangerous dispute. Sometimes rival pontificates had
been established for reasons of political expediency, sometimes
because of the shocking morals of those who had self-
interestedly eased themselves on to the papal throne, sometimes
because of the corruption of the curia. Whatever the direct
causes, the first of such rivalries may be said to be the simultaneous pontificates of Calixtus I and Hippolytus, who were elected
in the year 217. Hippolytus was an extreme puritan and an
extreme snob who accused Calixtus of being no more than a
morally dubious slave who had risen by way of personal
machinations. He caused himself to be irregularly elected and
consecrated as the first anti-pope so that he might wage doc-
trinal war with Calixtus; but his theological rage did neither
him nor his adversary any good, for both of them were sent by
the emperor Maximinus to penal servitude in the Sardinian
mines in 235. However, in that first rivalry may be marked the
tiny fissure that was to widen into the Great Schism that lasted
from 1378 to 1417.

The bridging of the schism was not the only task the council of Constance set itself. The reformation of the whole policy of the church was, from a temporal point of view, of even greater importance. Abuse of riches, corruption of the curia, the revolt of the Hussites in Bohemia, the ostentatious magnificence of the papal court, the question of whether the Greek or Roman branches of the church should be politically supreme—these matters, and many others, were the urgent concern of the common people. That concern had reached its climax under the popular leadership of John Wyclif in England, Jan Hus in Bohemia, and Gerard Groot in the Netherlands, all of whom, in their different ways, demanded reforms that would lead to greater simplicity in the leadership of the christian faith. The reforms were not forthcoming from the council's deliberations—indeed Wyclif was condemned as an heretic and Jan Hus was burned at the stake—and in fact were not implemented until after Spanish and German mercenaries plundered Rome in 1527, by which time the influence of the church had been drained almost to nothing by a succession of popes who were weak, cruel, or like Alexander VI (Rodrigo Borgia), ridden with secular megalomania and lacking even belief in the faith of which he was head. The four popes who in their turn succeeded the Borgia instituted the reforms that were to restore the cohesion of the church and from which, after the sack of Rome, began to emerge the ever-increasing forces of the Reformation and counter-Reformation.

The Renaissance, considered as a revival of thought and learning, was a reaction against the influence of the barbaric middle ages and their crumbling empires. The classical traditions of Greece and Rome had been lost with the fall of Byzantium; but with the diminishing influence of the church caused by the schism a new interest in those traditions began. The whole of Europe was in fact afire with the spirit of reform, with the impulse of discovery such as that which set the face of the Genoese sailor Christopher Columbus toward what he thought to be the Indies, and with a burgeoning knowledge of the nature of the world. Henceforth christian men were to press the claims of the individual human spirit against the assumption of temporal power by the church. They could point to the truth that the unity of the faith had been preserved by the common people, not by the disputatious papacy that had all but brought about its downfall. Their fiery spirit manifested itself in painting, in sculpture, in literature; in architecture, in astronomy, astrology, mathematics and exploration; in law and music and medicine. Scarcely any of the fields of cultural and scientific learning were left unruffled by the impetus of the Renaissance, though the word itself, used to describe the era, did not come into common use for three hundred years.

The era, as I have said, is not to be bound by any arbitrary limits. The impetus, though violent and fiery, was everywhere hindered by the slowness of communications in those days. Long before 1414 Italian artists, sculptors, astronomers, and mathematicians had felt the stirrings of new impulses; and long after 1527 the revival of interest in the classical traditions were still spreading to Spain, Germany, and France. Also, both before and after those convenient dates, there was a mingling with other influences. So the Renaissance should be seen as a purlieus of influence most sharply defined in the last years of the 15th and first of the 16th centuries but gradually dispossessing itself of medievalism before and as gradually submitting to the dominance of the Reformation after.

It should also be seen as a time when reverence toward the specialist in a particular field of learning was waning. Such a man as Chaucer, who died about 1400 and was a prominent public figure as a magistrate, diplomat, and court story-teller, would have been lauded for his ability as an efficient official and court entertainer; also, in the case of those of his works that filtered through to the public, for his astringent evaluation of human nature. But that was specialization; and although no one knows for certain the breadth of his learning, it seems improbable that his mind embraced much outside the fields of poetry and the civil service. And so it was with many other of the great figures of the Middle Ages. Roger Bacon, Thomas Aquinas, Dante, Giotto—these are names associated with one, or at most two, branches of activity or learning. There were few jacks-of-all-trades and no masters of them all. But with the Renaissance came men who saw the burnished fields of learning in panoramic array and whose intellects could stretch to grasp wider horizons than those confined within the narrow limits of a single art or science.

The obvious and greatest example of such a man is Leonardo, the breadth of whose vision had been unequalled since the greatest days of Greek culture, and whose grasp of all the natural sciences and achievements in the visual and plastic arts, in music, mathematics, and engineering, was phenomenal. His birth place, Vinci, in Tuscany, saw little of him after his childhood. His cities were Florence, where he served his apprenticeship as a painter, and Milan. He was no great traveller, and no christian either, in spite of the religious subject matter of many of his paintings, for his pantheistic vision was incapable of being confined within the limits of a single doctrine. And although he lived in the age of patronage when defection from the political faction of a patron could mean prison, torture or death, it is a measure of his genius that his complete lack of political loyalty went unmarked. He was at once a part of the sociological structure of the age and loftily independent of it, as is the way with geniuses.

The sociological structure and the political structure were of course inseparable. "Italy was then a country of petty sovereigns arrayed against each other. The larger republics, such as Florence and Venice, were filled with an insatiable desire to possess the smaller states of Genoa, Pisa, and Siena; for this they leagued themselves alternately with France and Germany. Both these countries had claims on Milan and Naples, and their contentions filled the whole century with a succession of wars and leagues, of treachery and rapine."[1] Compared with today's global strife those wars were tiny and bloodless. But in the limited confines of a city or district no doubt they seemed as cruel and terrifying, though they were fought with all the panoply of magnificence that matched the age. The petty meannesses of such military enterprises as the sack of Rome were disastrous for scholarship, and it is only because of the richness of that scholarship that so much has been preserved. As an example of the losses one might instance the lifetime's work of Antonio Valdo, a great traveller who had just completed his *magnum opus* on the peoples of Bohemia and saw his manuscript consumed in the flames of a fire lit by the looters to cook their meat on while he, starving, was crucified to the door of his own workroom.[2] The cruelty of individual rulers also was noteworthy. Giovanni Maria of the dynasty of the Visconti, who succeeded to the Dukedom of Milan in the 15th century, contrasts bleakly with the Sforza, who succeeded the Visconti as rulers of the province. Confusion and struggle continued throughout Giovanni's reign. "The condition of the city was lamentable. Peace and order were destroyed, and the names of Guelf and Ghibelline were heard again in the streets, inflaming household against household and awakening the horrors of civil war. The Duke made no attempt to rule for himself. His only share in the government was the execution of State prisoners, whom he caused to be torn to pieces, under his own eyes, by dogs trained for the purpose. The extraordinary passion for dogs, together with the hatred of humankind . . . had become an extravagant ferocity in this degenerate member of the race. The story of Milan during his reign is like some dreadful dream, in which, when sleep has fallen on the incessant riots and fighting, through the darkness of the night stalk the awful figures of the maniac Prince, gloating in his sport, and his huntsman, Squarcia Giramo, beside him, with their terrible hounds in leash, on the scent of human blood. The Duke's appetite for blood was rewarded with Dantesque fitness. He died in 1412, suffocated in his own blood in the precincts of the palace, under the daggers of three Milanese nobles, who had sworn to rid the world of a monster, and his body, lying in its blood in the Cathedral, whither it had been carried and left alone by the general horror, had for its only pall blood-red roses strewn upon it by a harlot".[3]

The confusion and struggle, if not Giovanni's canine megalomania, continued long after his death. But the age, as by now, I hope, is clear, was an age of confusion, of brilliance, of discovery and recovery, of pomp and corruption, squalor and plague. Throughout the 15th century the renascent forces grew, carrying with them those influences of the Middle Ages that had not been swept away, and already anticipating, in some measure, the later forces of the Reformation that in turn, in the next century, were to become dominant. One could do worse than take as an analagous example of the confused struggle out of which Renaissance and Reformation formed the foundations of modern Europe, the building of Milan cathedral.

It was sponsored by Giovanni Visconti's father, Gian, the first Duke of Milan. His sponsorship was in part an atonement for bloodily usurping the dukedom, in part a monument to his own ambition to become ruler of the entire peninsula of Italy. Work began on it in 1386 and six years later the outer walls and interior pillars were completed. No one knows who submitted the design that the Duke presumably approved; but whoever it was disappeared from the scene very quickly, having handed over the execution of his plan to the Lombard guild of stonemasons. Among them there was apparently no personality strong enough to insist on interpreting the perfect balance of the Gothic design—or perhaps it was that that balance which, in the finest examples, was never over-elaborated to the point of fussiness, displeased the less austere notions of men who lived south of the Alps. At all events, they seem to have had little faith in their own ideas and turned instead to foreign architects for inspiration. Since all these differed on what should be done and each intrigued to get his own notions adopted, the conflict soon developed to a stage where destruction rather than construction was going on. One French builder declared the fabric unsafe and began to pull it down. His action was disputed and he was forced to put everything back as he found it, after which he was dismissed without fee and sent back to France. Similar conflicts developed between the Lombards and the Dutch and German architects. There were innumerable meetings of the Council of the Fabric. They were spread over many years and nothing was achieved at them except noisy argument and table banging. The work, however, proceeded. Sons succeeded fathers in the generations of masons, and gradually the great cathedral grew. But the inspiration that should have flowed between design and execution was all to conspicuous by its absence. Consciousness of the poverty of ideas was manifested by the wealth of ornamentation; but turrets, statues, and frets by the thousand cannot conceal the lack of guiding genius. Once the roof was on and the monstrous wedding-cake cupola added, work stopped and started and stopped again. These fits and starts were to be spread over nearly four centuries until the lacy confection was completed for the crowning of Napoleon in 1815. By that time restoration and addition had left little of the handiwork of the 15th-century builders—which was perhaps just as well; but those who followed them were no better and only added more and more tracery to the façade and more pinnacles and statues to the roof. The restlessness of the design of the cathedral is indeed a reminder in marmoreal form of the restlessness of the age in which it was begun and of the confusion that rent Italy in those days.

On 16 May 1509 Louis XII of France, leading seven companies of his best troops, entered Milan by the south gate. Two days earlier he and his expeditionary force had stormed the western defences of the state of Venice, which lay along the river Adda twenty miles to the east of Milan, and the Venetians were now in full rout. They had been pursued to the gate of their capital city by Louis's equally disorderly but numerically superior Milanese troops; and it was that rout that Louis was celebrating with a display of splendour he hoped would please the people of his duchy of Milan.

In fact it gave them no great pleasure. Epidemics of enteric and plague had broken out in the city two weeks earlier and all assemblies held the threat of infection. But there was a lively attendance all the same. Louis, who was busily earning his sobriquet Father of the People, was known to be kindly disposed in the matter of taxes; and he had already remitted his dues from the city in the cause of charity to the hospitals that housed the poor and now were additionally crowded with the sick. Also, nobody cared to act churlishly toward a king, even a king of an officially enemy country. He might easily have healing powers, and in any case his triumphal entry justified bibbing in the taverns earlier in the day than usual. Before eight in the morning crowds had arrived from outlying villages to mingle with the Milanese, and, confident in the prophylactic power of wine, were rolling into and out of the taverns and streets and converging on the immense square before the cathedral. There, there was plenty to amuse them and space to contain thirty thousand. A contemporary triptych recording the scene shows that the masons who were supposed to be working on the west side of the cathedral had started a quail-fight and were taking wagers on the birds, which were spurred with brass and no doubt had been forcibly fed on garlic to arouse their wrath; an angry priest has driven a puppeteer from the doorway of the cathedral and the man is scuttling round the square carrying his dolls and accompanied by a horde of children advising him on the selection of another venue for his performance; and itinerant scriveners, wine-sellers, fortune-tellers, lawyers, doctors, jesters and minstrels are all bustling about the great piazza in search of what business they can find before the arrival of the king.

The dramatic element of Louis's entry into Milan had been well secured. The heralds trumpeting his approach toward the city along the Via Pavia were followed at mid-morning by more heralds and a troop of cavalry attending upon the king's seneschal, riding a splendidly caparisoned horse. The seneschal, armoured at the knees, breast, and shoulders and helmeted in brass, wears also a short blue surcoat and looks impressive as he sits his horse beneath one of the triumphal arches that have been erected along the main Pavian way. The French artist who painted the scene shows him giving his orders to a group of *aides-de-camp* who listen attentively on bended knees and grasp lances carrying the king's gonfalon. It is clear that, when they have heard the orders, the *aides* will hurry round the city telling everyone what the seneschal says about general behaviour, where they should assemble, how much space to leave in the cathedral for the king and his troops to attend mass, and so on.

And at noon or thereabouts came the climax of the king's arrival. A 16th-century account of the occasion mentions the magnificence of his dress and the superb diamond he wore in his ermine-and-velvet cap; also that his tunic was "padded in the Spanish fashion to resemble armour and his sword prankt with rare jewels".[4] He was preceded by ratcatchers with terriers and falconers with hawks to deal with anything pestiferous that might cross his path, and by a posse of youths scattering saffron flowers to sweeten the city's foetid air. Musicians played festive music on trumpets and serpents; almoners distributed meat pies baked in the king's field kitchens to the beggars selected by the seneschal; and nearly four hundred scrofulous persons awaited the king's touch at the last triumphal arch on the route to the cathedral. He touched them all—spending, a contemporary pedant says, "one hour and the 29th part of a second hour"[5] on his healing gesture—and remarked on the need for more physicians in Milan. His seven companies of household troops, following him in parade order, had been accoutred by the finest Milanese armourers and their embossed casques and breastplates glinted in the sun. Their banners were of fine silk and made a proud pattern against the brazen sky.

All this splendour aroused enough enthusiasm to please the king, who later remarked that Milan was "a pretty city whose people commended themselves to my care".[6] It also entertained a small boy of eight years who watched from an upper window of a house in the Via dei Rovelli, which was on the main route of the kingly procession to the cathedral. His name was Gerolamo Cardano.

I

1501–1509

It may perhaps seem strange that the boy was watching
wanly—and indeed he looked pale and sad, he tells us so himself[1]—while the splendid cavalcade wound its way through the
outskirts of the city toward the piazza. Surely he should have
been down there in the streets, shouting huzzahs as the ratcatchers and the falconers and the youths with their posies of
flowers gave way to the heralds, the musicians, and the
armoured soldiers? Surely he should have been scampering
about with those other children whose concern was to find the
banished puppeteer a new theatre of operations? Should he not
have been seeking some spot where, though pressed by throngs
on every side, he could peer between some tall man's legs or beg
for a pick-a-back on to some kindly citizen's shoulders so that he
too could doff his cap as the king passed by? Why, when every
able man, woman, and child had by now overcome such hesita-
tion as may have been felt at the thought of possible infection,
and had been enticed into the streets by the glamorous excuse to
set aside work for the day—why should the lad be incarcerated
there on that upper floor, a spectator only and never a partici-
pant in the event that he was to remember for so long and
which was, in its fateful way, to reshape his life? Two answers
spring clearly to mind : that he was being punished for some
childish misdemeanor by being forbidden the gay streets, or that
he was ill. And indeed both explanations could so exactly have
fitted the pattern of his life up to that day that either could have
served. He was himself to remark in his reminiscences, written
nearly seventy years later, "sickness of body, and gloom of mind
in consequence of some injustice in my tutelage, were my daily
companions".[2] As indeed they were.

This time it was illness that was the cause of his being able to be only a detached spectator of the hurly-burly and the ceremony, aloft and wistful in his parents' shabby lodgings; but mercifully it was not the plague of the Black Death that for nearly two more centuries was to remain the sickening scourge of Europe, and which, as I have said, was at that very time dangerously evident in certain quarters of the city; nor was it the lesser but still frequently killing curse of enteric which also had broken out. It was something much more childish, a simple stomach-ache—brought by the child upon himself—, that had started the trouble. Scarcely, one might think, worth much comment. But since it was to lead to, among other things, the naming and baptism of the boy, and in large part to the decision, taken that day of the entry of Louis into Milan, which was so largely to influence his future, something more than a cursory mention is justified.

The boy was born, unhonoured, unwanted, but triumphant over the early efforts of his mother to abort him, at 6.30 on the evening of 24 September 1501. His parents were not married. His mother, whose name was Chiara Alberio, was the widow of a man of whom history says nothing except the manner of his death. That came about after a brawl in a tavern during a game of cards in which he had been cheating. Discovering that he was wearing a ring in which was set a mirror that reflected the faces of the cards being dealt, his opponents set about him, severed all the fingers of his right hand, branded him on the cheek, and flung him into the canal, where, being unable to swim, he drowned. Chiara came of a family, the Micheria, who appear to have been learned, penniless, and nomadic, so that one finds traces of them in Tuscany, in Sardinia, in Rome, in Pompeii; but traces so sparse that they cumulate only into an itinerary, never a history. She married Alberio when she was thirty and had three sons, Tommaso, Catalina, and Joanni; though it is by no means certain whether Alberio was the father. She was a woman apparently much in demand. "The number of her lovers", Gerolamo Cardano says in an unguarded moment, "approached the licentious."[3] It is possible that one or more of these, or even Gerolamo's own father, Fazio, sired them upon her. It is of little account. They died in 1502 during a virulent outbreak of plague, and the dynasty of Cardano nearly died with them, for the wet-nurse who was suckling Gerolamo also caught the plague and died of it and only by the determination of his physical resistance could she have failed to convey it to her charge.

Although he was to write wistfully—indeed somewhat self-pityingly—in his memoirs of his sickliness as a child, there can be no doubt that physically he was a very resilient little boy, while mentally he was precisely the opposite in that his lively mind was capable of a high degree of absorption of knowledge. Both characteristics were inherited from his father.

Fazio Cardano was by profession a geometer. But although the study of geometry was revered it was not a profession that could bring the student an income except by way of patronage. People have no material use for theorems even though they should pierce the mysteries of the universe. Law and medicine, however, are studies that can elucidate the problems of social intercourse and physical well-being, both of immense concern to mankind, and it was in these fields that Fazio wandered with most financial success. He had considerable skill in both of them; but in that society that paid so much respect to dynastic inheritance he was able to attract a widening clientéle by his claim to collateral association with the high-born Castillione family and descent from a brother of Godfrey of Milan, who was elected pope as Celestine IV in 1241 but died a few months later without being consecrated. Had he not been so feckless in character, Fazio might well have become a wealthy man; but he was for ever being overcome by accumulated debts piled up by Chiara's family and numerous other parasites who attached themselves to his household; and he was for ever discovering with other-wordly credulity that the dependants he had supposed in dire straits were in fact merely afflicted with cupidity. In consequence he became irascible in temper and withdrew more and more into a world of scholarship. Physically, he was unprepossessing. He had very pale eyes and a skull that was misshapen because he had fallen on it in youth and had had some splinters of bone removed from it by a drunken surgeon; as a result hair grew upon it only in separate tufts and he always wore a hat to conceal the deformed and scarecrow appearance of his head. When being barbered he allowed the barber to cut only one tuft at a time, believing that he would catch cold if left uncapped for more than a few minutes. He was round-shouldered through excessive poring over books, and completely toothless. He lacked teeth because, he said, he had once dispensed a draught to cure a choleric stomach and by mistake had put some corrosive substance into the mixture— "Fortune made my tongue detect the harshness of the flavour before swallowing, and I ejected the noxious thing; but my teeth spat out with it, loosened in the gums by the acid, and rattled like dice upon the floor".[4] Unprepossessing outwardly, he suffered also from palpitations of the heart and constant indigestion; but these defects certainly did not shorten his life, for he lived eighty years, having been born in 1445 and buried in 1525.

When Gerolamo was born, Chiara and Fazio were in the midst of one of the countless domestic upheavals round which their feckless lives turned. There had been a quarrel the cause of which, among so many, it is now impossible to determine, and she had fled from him in high dudgeon—by no means for the first time. Certainly her decision had been reinforced by the epidemic of plague which at that time—as so often in Renaissance days—was bringing about a general exodus from the city of Milan; but inoculated as she was by an earlier bubonic infection from which she had recovered, it is doubtful if the threat of sickness alone would have forced her flight. She was hardy in health and by nature indomitable; and because indomitable also dominating and truculent—characteristics that accorded ill with Fazia Cardano's irascibility. Hence the frequent outbursts and separations.

Chiara's destination was the home of her sister Margarita in Pavia, twenty miles to the south. There is no record of how she accomplished the journey, but in her state of advanced pregnancy one hopes she did not have to walk. However she got there, she arrived, according to Gerolamo, who presumably had it from her during one of the autobiographical narratives with which mothers enlighten their children, on 15 August 1501. She and her sister were of similar temperaments, though Margarita was, some said, the worse a harridan for having remained a spinster; and it seems unlikely that the time during which her sister harboured with her was any more peaceful than that which Chiara had recently endured with Fazio. No doubt the mother-to-be forced upon her sister bitter tirades about her condition; she certainly left record that she neither liked children nor wanted any more and that she had attempted an abortion in the fourth month of her pregnancy by drinking a potion of colewort, tamarisk root, burnt barleycorns, and wormwood. Understandably this potion failed to do anything but make her vomit, and for five more months her bitterness was manifested by her increasing tendency to put the blame, first, upon Fazio, and, after she had left him, upon anyone else who chanced to be within quarrelling distance. She was not at that time an endearing woman. Nor was she even a physically attractive one, for she was short, fat, and bloated; and she was given to hypocritical outbursts of unctuous piety between her sulks and rages. But as compensatory virtues she had wit and the indefinable charm often given to women of little beauty.

The child was born after a protracted labour of three days. The midwife pessimistically told Margarita that she feared "The child must surely be a monster when at last he puts upon the world, for devils have had easy time to work their evils while he is thus delayed in darkness".[5] The baby was not a monster, but he was frail and silent; and the nurse, muttering to Margarita that he could not live more than an hour, instructed her to warm a bath of wine and meanwhile lay the child by while she attended to Chiara. When the wine was warm she put the baby in it and he immediately began to bellow lustily. He lived for another seventy-five years in spite of the midwife's gloomy prognostication. The time of his birth—6.30 in the evening and the date—24 September—formed an astrological conjunction that Gerolamo was later to blame for a great many of his troubles.

Those troubles began almost at once. The nurse and Gerolamo's three half-brothers (or brothers, as the case may be), who evidently were also being sheltered by Margarita, caught the plague and within a year had died; and Gerolamo also fell sick of it in a mild way. But, probably because Chiara had transmitted to him some of her natural resistance, he recovered and

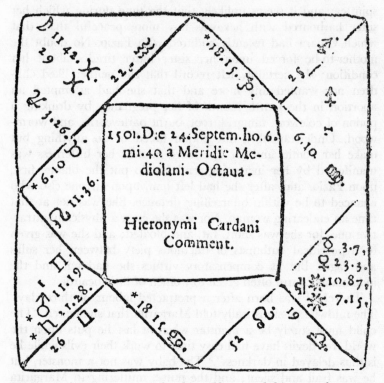

1501. D:e 24. Septem. ho. 6. mi. 40 à Meridie Mediolani. Octaua.

Hieronymi Cardani Comment.

Cardano's horoscope, cast by himself, caused him much appre hension

had no inheritance from the illness except some unpleasant scrofulous patches on his face. These later developed into five
typical plague-warts—one on the end of his nose, one on his
forehead, one on each cheek, and one on the chin. But in his
childhood there were many other cruel strokes of fate in the
form of illness. Chiara was unable, or perhaps unwilling, to feed
him and he was put out to a succession of wet-nurses who
accepted the fees paid but, either because of the fear of con-
tracting the plague themselves or because they were continually
drunk or whoring, neglected him until he was a swollen-bellied
starveling. In that state he was discovered in the foul hovel of
the latest of the nurses by the housekeeper of a nobleman, Isadoro dei Resti, who was employing Fazio as his adviser in a

legal matter connected with the senate. Isadoro compassionately took the child into his own luxurious home in Pavia and found for him a foster mother who was lactifically efficient and unafraid of contagion. But it was a long engagement with the spectre of starvation, and only when the child was three years old was he at last weaned and returned to Chiara.

She, it must be said to her credit, now began to show some signs of affection for him; but her domestic circumstances were as variable as ever they had been. Sometimes she seems to have been living in the poorest of lodgings, sometimes in comparatively ample homes. Invariably Margarita was with her; and sometimes Fazio also. The cities of Pavia and Milan embraced and discarded them according to fortune. It is not hard to deduce the reason for the continual disruption of the Cardano household: landlords probably had great difficulty in securing their rent, and compassionate friends who sheltered the family must have grown weary of the perpetual quarrels that went on. In that atmosphere of disharmony Gerolamo himself came in for a good deal of beating; but he seems not to have resented it, for he remarks in his reminiscences, "Perchance a touch of the whip did me no harm".[6] Maltreatment, though, may well have made him brood upon the injustices of life; it certainly made him an introspective child, for he was afraid to pursue any of the normal extrovert activities of children in case he should incur more wrath. The refuges of contemplation were, however, of great comfort to him. This being one of the great eras when the intellect was paramount in importance, when academic debates on the nature of the universe and of humanity's place within it were ordinary social diversions in the home, he was at all times encouraged to extend the gropings of his own mind. He frequently sought to analyse his own condition, to study the causes of his own misfortune. And even discountenancing as just the frequent whippings dealt out by his parents and aunt, his misfortunes were numerous. He was what we should today call accident-prone. He had only to sit upon the threshold of the Cardano lodgings for a stone to work loose from the parapet and fell him into bleeding unconsciousness. More than once he fell down flights of steps—on one occasion letting fly a hammer he was carrying which thereupon described an arc and landed on his skull as he tumbled to the foot; and he had only to cross a canal for the rail of the bridge to give way and let him down into the water. Since astrology was then a greatly revered science and he was constantly in the company of adults who talked of it, he attributed his ill-fortune to the influence of the stars and resigned himself to the certainty that there would be no change of fate for him until they shifted in their courses to a more favourable position. In that he was accepting a common theory; but that he did not accept it without question is shown by a comment he made in a letter written to a fellow student in 1519 : "It was very well for my father to wring his hands at the issue of fortune determined by the [heavenly] bodies on the houses where we set our homes; but I recall thinking that the distance was very great for such an issue to be made, for might not the sun shine on Cathay when rain fell upon Padua? And if the biggest star of all could not stretch its warmth thus far, how could the smaller ones seem to malign from such a height? Now I know I was in error; but it was a childish curiosity and not without the gleanings of a cynic".[7]

The lesser inflictions of Gerolamo's childhood included tasks that would more suitably have been given to a beast of burden. From the age of five his father made him carry increasingly large loads of the legal and medical books he needed when visiting his patrons. The boy had strapped to his back a pannier into which books were stuffed; he had also to carry books in his arms and occasionally upon his head. "From time to time as we walked the streets my father would command me to stop while he opened a book and, using my head as a table, read some long passage, prodding me the while with his foot to keep still if I wearied of the great weight."[8]

Just as, upon his return to her from the beneficent succour of Isadoro dei Resti, Chiara manifested a change of heart toward her unwanted son, so, after several years of treating Gerolamo as an unpaid labourer, Fazio also changed his attitude. His acquaintances noted it, but were at variance as to the cause. One said it was brought about by a dream which Fazio had interpreted as a warning from astral planes; another thought that the geometer had shrewdly realized that the boy was likely to be of greater use if he was treated with some consideration and not allowed to fall into a decline. Whatever the inspiration, Fazio undoubtedly began to treat the boy with comparative kindness. He lessened his burdens, included him in the mumbling conversations he carried on with himself as he shuffled about Milan in velvet gown and pantoufles, and occasionally took him into the houses of mathematicians, physicians, and lawyers to listen to their arguments.

It was one of these arguments, so fierce and prolonged, that led directly to the simple stomach-ache the after effects of which were to bring about Gerolamo's baptism, his incarceration in the upper room on the day of Louis's entry into Milan, and the thoughts that were to shape his career.

One day in April 1509 Fazio had an appointment to visit two elderly geometers who lived near the Palazzo della Ragione. They were to thrash out some new angular theorem that Fazio had formulated and it promised—and indeed proved—to be a long discussion. It was one of the occasions when Fazio was accompanied by Gerolamo, who was relatively lightly burdened with Fazio's manuscripts in which the theorem was notated, and who was taken by his father into the sanctum where the discussion was to be held. It was a chamber filled with fascinations for the child. Charts, manuscripts, books, globes, lamps, retorts, embryo mechanisms, strange jewels and mummified creatures, pelts, lumps of amber and agate jars, herbs, skins full of wine : there seemed at first to be no end to the infinite variety of things to be seen and examined. And indeed Gerolamo assures us that they were. "I spent above two hours inspecting and fondling these miraculous things, all filled with delight for a child of small years. The voices of my father and his companions, to which in other circumstances I should have been dutifully listening with my chin cupped in my hands, went droning on like bees in a garden where I was enticed by the flowers. I gave them no attention. They rose and fell, and I suppose changed in tone as this or that argument was countered with another. I was busily peering into every corner, gazing with wonder on instruments I dared not touch, on jewels and stones that flamed with mystery. But at length, it seemed, I had examined all. My tongue was bursting with questions I dared not

ask, and my ears had long lost the process of the argument that
went on round the table." In short, the child became bored and
sought about for some new interest to occupy his lively mind.
Unseen, he slipped away from the room and found himself in
another, where, on a refectory table stood a great bowl of very
fine grapes. These he began to eat and continued until he had
eaten several bunches, when he guiltily arranged the remainder
so that the bowl still looked full. Later in the day this indulgence brought him an attack of colic and much vomiting.

Only the day before news had been heard of a case of enteric*
on the other side of the city. Fazio took Gerolamo's symptoms to be those of the dreaded fever and was startled into
apprehension about the boy's health. And, since in those days
men still saw the consequences of their sins of commission and
omission in literal ways, he may well have also felt the twinges
of a guilty conscience. At all events, being temporarily in funds
from a fee he had earned by unravelling a complex point of
Roman law for the senate, he summoned doctors whose knowledge he could pool with his own to effect a cure. Together,
holding vinegar-soaked kerchiefs to their faces to lessen the risk
of infection, they had their consultation round the boy's bed.
Purges, poultices, and surgery were all suggested as remedies,
Gerolamo recalls in his reminiscences, and adds sharply, "A
rumbling gut is no cause to be cut up alive, even for a child
who has stolen the fruit that caused it, and I began my exer-
tions to leap from the bed, pale and fevered though I was; but
the grave physicians thus thought I was tortured by greater pain
and approaching death and must at once be seen by a priest to
ensure my safe conduct to paradise".[9] This startled Fazio into
recalling that the boy had never been named or baptized and
that a name and holy unction had better be bestowed quickly or
he, Fazio, might find hindrance with his own heavenly journey
when the time came.[10]

Having given their advice and taken their fees the doctors
departed, leaving Fazio with his new problem: that of a name
for the boy. Overcome with remorse, he decided that the name

---

* Another name for typhoid fever. In those days there was much
confusion between typhus and typhoid, both of which were prevalent, and
which usually received no more specific nomenclature than "fever".

should perpetuate that of a saint so that candles could be lighted and prayers offered, and in those obeisances some of the responsibility shifted from his own shoulders. But which saint? It was not a choice lightly to be made. In the whole calendar of those canonized only guidance or inspiration could light upon the one proper to the case and the ocassion. He told Chiara that he was about to make some visits of importance and set off to call on various friends and acquaintances who might be relied upon for their advice. But he appears to have been disappointed in their suggestions, which, he said, were "not proper to the special case". Perplexed, he continued his ambulation, his head bent forward, his staff tapping upon the ground, until, wearying, he rested on a bench in the grounds of a hospice between the Pavian and Vercelline gates. The hospice was dedicated to Saint Gerolamo, who had been a Latin scholar and translator of the bible in the 5th century. But in spite of his pause in the garden the saint's name made no impression on him, and he set off home without his problem having been solved. On approaching the Via de Rovelli, he says, he was "Suddenly struck by violent lightnings in the head", and these seem to have illuminated the memory of the name of the man in whose house he was presently staying, Gerolamo Ermenulfo. That he had just come from one Gerolamo's garden and was making his way back to the house of another seemed to him to have divine meaning. He fell upon his knees in the street and prayed for intercession on the boy's behalf, striking at the same time a bargain with the spirit of Saint Gerolamo, to whom he generously offered to dedicate the boy's life. That done, he returned home, told Chiara his decision, and sent her and Margarita for a priest while he sat at his son's bedside.[11]

When the priest arrived he found the boy tranquil and with the internal pains greatly diminished. That was perhaps not surprising, considering that it was now more than twenty-four hours since his feast of stolen fruit. The priest, however, after sharply reproving Fazio for having wickedly neglected to have his son baptized, said that the boy's recovery was due to the intervention of God, who thus had signified that baptism should take place immediately and expensively, with Fazio making repentance in both monetary and spiritual ways. Thus rebuked,

2—DC

Fazio went to the confessional, accepted his penance, received absolution, and arranged for the ceremony.

In those days, baptism was no simple matter of a brief ceremony at which the priest dedicates the child to the service of God by naming him as directed by the godparents and marking upon his forehead, with a finger dipped in font water, a simple cross. Any priest worth the name insisted on total immersion in a tank filled with the holy water of the Jordan. The water was imported across the Mediterranean by the merchants who bought it from water-leaders who in turn had transported it across the sands of Arabia in water-skins borne by caravans of camels. The opportunities for sharp practice on the part of the merchants must have been numerous and were probably irresistible, and no doubt much baptismal water came from sources less holy than the Jordan; but in such matters belief is all important, and it was the belief of the most earnest priests that the water was holy and that only complete immersion in it could bring complete baptismal holiness. So Gerolamo, still weak from the effects of the colic, was wrapped in cloaks and taken to the baptistery, where the full ceremonial rite was performed. He was to remember for years that, "The water was warm but of a slimy disposition, with mollusca clinging to the stone walls, and when all the prayers had been said I was made dry with ferns and linen napkins and returned to my bed".

It was scarcely surprising that immersion in a bath of unwholesome, if holy, water—of which no doubt some was swallowed—should have retarded his recovery. His fever returned, and for two weeks he had periods of delirium, blackness of the tongue, and continual intestinal disorders. On this occasion Fazio himself treated him with herbs and strong wine, which in due course reduced the fever and brought the boy to a state of convalescence in which, though terribly weak from lack of food, some of the colour had returned to his cheeks and he was able to rise from his bed for a while each day. And thus we find him on 16 May, wanly peering down on the Via dei Rovelli, along which the rearguard of the gorgeous procession has at last passed, and the crowds with it, so that the street is now empty of all save the blistering midday sunlight, an emaciated dog or two that scuttled to safety when the first tuckets were heard in the distance, and a leprous beggar who had been whipped and prodded to the distance deemed safe for a pariah and now returned to scavenge among maloderous corners for pickings of discarded food. The scent of saffron has long died in the foetid air; the heat sweeps down; dust raised by the multitude of horses' hooves settles slowly on roof, pediment, and threshold. The splendour is marked now only by the sound of the throng as it moves toward the cathedral, where Louis and his entourage will hear mass and give thanks for his petty victory.

Gerolamo tells us his thoughts[12] as he looked down; but they are thoughts recalled over nearly seventy years and the bulk of them are too obviously influenced by hindsight. Many subtractions must be made. One thought, however, need not be subtracted : "I had had enough and enough of law; its books, by my experience, were heavy and its conclusions unsatisfactory, for they rarely brought to an end the arguments of social custom, and however the outcome of a single argument absolute justice was never to be proved, the nature of the litigants making such proof impossible, both desiring victory for selfish as well as just reasons. It was a pursuit of ends through the passages of a maze where the key was lost and buried and the exit not to be arrived at, only by circuits of words in which all who read and heard them were like [wise] lost in littler but no less sinister mazes. Numbers I thought greatly of for what they could prove, and Euclid also for what he could say of the world and set it down in plane and prove that too; and medicine which is the concern of all, that the functions of their bodies may be discovered and understood—the choler of the brain, why it rises in certain heats and is to be withdrawn downward, sometimes to a place cut by a surgeon, and why the hands and feet of some, like my own, are cold until dawn even abed. Also the affliction of the leper and how it comes about and what is to be done for it." That thought, divorced from its prolix and flamboyant context, of which much is the muttering of an old man, gives the clue as to some of the courses along which he thought to direct his life on that hot day in Milan. Arithmetic, geometry, medicine—the roads widen before him in his precocious imagination.

2

1514 – 1518

Gerolamo's was a typically Renaissance intellect: it was closed to nothing and there was little that failed to excite its interest. Lacking Leonardo da Vinci's art and genius, he nevertheless was, in the fertility of his mind, somewhat similar—a miniature, as it were, of the mighty creator. It may be inferred from what I have quoted of his recollections that he was also a charmless and precocious child, for it is unusual at the age of eight to moralize about one's path in life. But the hindsight of old age gives shape to thoughts that in childhood are vague. Doubtless his decision to discard law and turn to the precise sciences of arithmetic and geometry, and the compassionate one of medicine, was subliminal. He had probably been moved by emotion at the sight of the leprous beggar rather than by reasoning. But he is so insistent that "At that day's end my life had swung upon its swivel" that we must accept his word.

Swung though it may have, however, it naturally for some years followed the course of ordinary learning. Fazio taught him the reading and writing of Italian and Latin—then the only tongue used by the learned—, and the rudiments of geometry, astronomy, astrology, and arithmetic. Nobody taught him hypochondria or self-pity: they were inherent in his character; and accidents and minor ailments so frequently afflicted him that perhaps it is not surprising that he could scarcely go through a day without believing something to be wrong with him and without suffering the mockery of his friends for so believing. So, gradually, "as much as it was permitted to me", he tells us gloomily, "I lived to myself; and, in some hope of future things, despised the present". It seems a joyless way of living for a child, and again some allowance must be made for the exaggerations of hindsight. But there is no doubt of his eagerness and ability to learn; or, indeed, of his ambition to leave his name to the world. "I desire to defend myself from obscurity", he wrote in a letter accompanying a manuscript that he sent to a friend in Como, Agostino Lavizario. The letter went on to explain that in his manuscript he had developed an equation of Jabir ibn Haijan's,* "So that by my method I teach how and why, the latitude and longitude of two places or stars being known, their true distance from each other may be calculated". Gerolamo was then twelve years old and it would be interesting to be able to comment on his geometrical theory; but unfortunately Lavizario lost the manuscript and only the precocious covering letter survived. Cardano's name also survives, which surely would have pleased him. However unwittingly, it is recalled by every aficianado of the modern motor-car who refers to the cardanshaft and its universal joint—a mechanism invented by Gerolamo during a period of intense mechanical creativeness, when his notebooks reveal activities that almost vie with Leonardo's in their scope and ingenuity.

That, however, lay ahead.

The days of Gerolamo's youth pass with ordered vigour. Seemingly, no hour, no minute, is claimed by idleness. He rises at nine in the morning "when the rheum is gone from the dawn and its chill",[1] and is summoned at once by Fazio to begin the day's studies. For an hour or more he writes his Latin exercises while Fazio irascibly corrects him and stoops over his own books. Asides from the old man lead Gerolamo to make notes : witchcraft, unicorns, the circulation of the blood, the constitution of the senate, horoscopes, games with cards and dice, cures for warts and impotence, the ways of animals and birds, architecture, ballistics : these and a hundred other things are to be investigated in the libraries of scholars. With Fazio he pays a visit to Leonardo, then (1514) at the height of his fame, and Gerolamo listens attentively while the two old men discuss a problem of geometry. "My father's reputation as a scholar was such that he was consulted by superior persons", he remarks

---

* Sometimes called Gaber. He was an 8th-century Arabic alchemist who wrote treatises on astronomy.

with a ducal snobbishness that ill becomes him.[2] He is as concerned with the architecture of a spider's web as with the arguments over the cupola of Milan cathedral. He is enthralled by the Christmas fair at Venice, to which he makes the long journey with Fazio, who is attending a conference of jurisconsults at the end of 1515. The merchants in the harbour fascinate him with their markets and their noisome bargaining over the price of pepper, saffron, ginger, nutmeg, malmsey, oil, and figs, while the huge Flanders galleys stand at the quays and there is a tumult when one of them is sunk by a mutinous crew. "Full learning makyth me full", he observes with little originality but with laudable intention to note the humdrum as well as the startling.[3]

Back in Milan in the spring of 1516 he notes for the first time his love of music. In a single day he hears mass five times for the pleasure of the sound of the unaccompanied voices. When the fortunes of the family are on the wane and they are in poor and tumbledown lodgings he invites himself to the homes of friends to hear concerts of viols and recorders; with the waxing of the fortunes he himself becomes the host and madrigal singers and lutenists sing and play in the evenings. Fazio was an accomplished keyboard player, Margarita was not without talent as a singer, and Chiara added words which Gerolamo refers to with implications of bawdiness. There is a great deal of pleasure to be found in music. It is a pleasure that is to last him all his life Painting also. He evidently visited the convent of Santa Maria delle Grazie when *The Last Supper* was still in its glowing splendour on the wall of the refectory, for in 1532 he was to remark that "the composition seems blurred and colourless compared with what I remember of it when I saw it as a boy".[4] And indeed, as all the world now knows, Leonardo's experimental use of oils was to prove the great fresco's ruin. The repeated "restorations" of later artists have practically obliterated the master's work, and the print we know so well is of course a reproduction of the copy of Leonardo's pupil Marco d'Oggiono. Had Gerolamo known that the Dominicans were to cut a door through Leonardo's masterpiece into their kitchen, and that Napoleon's horses were to be stabled in the refectory and kick their heels at the fresco, he might have felt outraged as well as puzzled at the fading of the picture.

All the days of his youth, then, are filled with learning and active leisure. He practices on the spinet, the recorder, and the viol, and becomes proficient in all of them—or so he tells us himself, and we should perhaps make allowances for vanity as well as snobbishness. At sixteen he can converse in Latin; but his father, possibly with the object of quelling his vainglory, persists in giving him menial tasks to perform. "I still had to carry his bag and fretted at the weight of books; but he would not relent in humiliating me thus, nor in striking me if my protests became too loud".[5] In spite of this treatment, however, he revered Fazio; and the only storm between them whirls about the question of Gerolamo's proper education. He is sensitive to the contempt he imagines is cast upon him for his bastardy (though he never reproaches his parents for it) and longs to leave the company of his father's circle in Milan and become a student at Fazio's *alma mater* in Pavia. This is forbidden him because Fazio finds him too useful as amanuensis and unpaid porter. There are innumerable family quarrels in consequence. Chiara's affection for her unwanted son had so increased that she staunchly takes his part in his continual pleading for further education, which Fazio as continually rejects. Some of these quarrels lead to physical violence. On one occasion Fazio strikes Chiara about the shoulders with his staff and she falls with a cry, striking her head against a table. Margarita in turn sets about the old man and drives him from the room. Chiara lies bleeding, and foaming at the mouth with rage. In the midst of this vulgar display Gerolamo shouts that he will take himself off to a monastery and conceal himself from the tempestuous world within a monk's cowl. Margarita shouts in turn that they will be well rid of him. Fazio returns, wringing his hands with remorse, to bathe Chiara's bleeding head and administer a sedative. Chiara, her feminine wiles suddenly alive to the advantage of her situation, feigns groaning unconsciousness for three hours. At the end of that time she whispers with convincing feebleness that only Gerolamo's happiness can restore her to life. Otherwise she is prepared, and prefers, to die. Fazio surrenders—is in fact only too glad to, since Margarita's evidence as a witness of his attack upon her sister can be turned to malicious purpose, and Margarita is a malicious woman. So ends the fracas that is to take Gerolamo to the university of Pavia.

He had of course to be sponsored and admitted and to await the beginning of the new academic year. All that would take time. He had also to nominate a subject for special study. Since Fazio drew a small hereditary stipend of a hundred crowns annually from the court of jurisconsults, and this hereditament would fall naturally to Gerolamo if he qualified as a stipendiary lawyer, the mercenary choice lay plain. Fazio was an old man of seventy-four and was already showing signs of feebleness, and by the time Gerolamo finished his studies would probably be dead. The hundred crowns at least offer an even financial keel to launch his life upon. But Gerolamo cared little for money and even less for the law, as he had already determined. There were further arguments of great heat in the Cardano household, and in the end the youth had his way. He would study medicine.

"I began immediately to assess the troubles of my own body", he says with the glee of the hypochondriac who enjoys bad health, "and to think what benefits I could confer on mankind by its study and cure." And he sets down his body's size, shape, and failings at that time—the first of many explorations and chartings that he pores over and wonders about as if they describe some island where treasure lies buried but is all hedged about with the diabolical snares of pain and imperfection. From that first exercise in physical cartography we learn that as a child he was fat and red, but that now, approaching nineteen, he has grown to his full height—"no more than that of any man", he says with disappointment, as if there were some special virtue in height—has a narrow chest and very small feet, a long neck and thin arms, fair hair and a beard dressed in the fashionable forked style. Of the outward manifestations of his physique, he is also displeased with his voice, which is loud and rasping. As for his inward troubles, he suffered, he says, from backache, toothache, headaches, poor circulation that kept his hands and feet permanently cold, the stone, difficulty in breathing, galloping of the heart, and an infection of the nipples that caused him to scratch constantly.[6]

This apparently unappealing youth, however, did not lack companions, male or female. He reports his first heterosexual experience as having been deliberately delayed until he was eighteen but he is not explicit as to the reason for the delay. Judging from the somewhat bizarre details of the union, he appears to have been curiously uncertain of the functions of the female genital organs. But he had of course so far made no study of anatomy. His medical experience was limited to hearing his father prescribe treatment for fevers. His decision in 1509 to take up medicine as a career was an emotional one, and he had not implemented it by any studies—mainly, no doubt, because there had been no opportunity, and medicine is a pursuit that of all things needs practical demonstration. At all events, his clinical interest in his own body and the cataloguing of its defects is the first record we have of his studentship of the art in which he was to become most famous.

Having now achieved his object in persuading Fazio to let him enter the world of learning, he sensibly set about providing himself with the necessary money. Indifferent though he might be toward wealth for its own sake, he had no illusions about the need for a certain amount of it at Pavia. He had no patron to pay his dues, and he was too familiar with the variations in Fazio's earnings, and the unpredictable demands upon them, to place any reliability on that source. The only stable wealth in the family was in the hands of one of Fazio's two nephews, Ottone Cantone, a collector of taxes whose riches had been acquired by gifts of property and cash made to him by wealthy men whose tax liabilities he had surreptitiously adjusted. Ottone thought very highly of his cousin Gerolamo, was older than him by some forty years, and had lived so riotously on his easily-gotten gains that he had hastened his own progress toward a tax-free world. On his deathbed he told Fazio that he wished to leave his fortune to Gerolamo—"Who worthily will be advantaged by its inheritance".[7] Fazio, however, possibly out of pique at having been ignored in the proposed will, refused it on Gerolamo's behalf, supporting the refusal with the pious reproach that the wealth was acquired dishonestly, which was true; but scarcely, one would have thought, a matter for reproach by Fazio, whose own morals were far from immaculate. Gerolamo laconically observes that Ottone having died intestate, "The riches went in their due course to Evangelista [Ottone's brother], who spent them on piety in the hermitage where he was a Franciscan monk."[8]

So he had to look elsewhere for the means to support himself while at the university. The search was not a difficult one. He had mastered arithmetic and the first six books of Euclid, was brilliant in dialectics, had a working knowledge of alchemy and astronomy, and was familiar with the principal philosophical works. In all those subjects he found pupils. He could also cast horoscopes, and for those too there were innumerable willing buyers—typical of their age in that they sought the enlightenment of astrology while still wallowing in the darker conjurations of necromancy. But most profitable of all was his skill in gambling. I say skill advisedly, for he played mainly at dice, in which it may seem that only chance is involved, since no skill can control the falling of the little cubes unless it be by palming or weighting them. His skill lay, however, not in any devious means of ordering his own success—doubtless he was well aware of the grim end to which Alberio had come—but in his ability to calculate his chances and bet accordingly. At first he recognized the ability only in a shadowy way; but gradually he came to realize that he could at least minimize his losses by placing his stakes cunningly. It occurred to him then that the machinations of "the Prince of fortune" might continually be counteracted by his own machinations. The fact that he often lost even when calculating his chances to what should have been his certain advantage, seemed to him to indicate only that he had not worked out the proper formulae; and he determined to do so. He was to discover, as most gamblers do, that the Prince of fortune is not so easily cheated; but his study of the subject was to lead to the propounding of the Laws of Probability as we know them today. Meanwhile, enjoying both a long run of luck and the advantage over his opponents that his calculations gave him, he flourished financially and was able to set aside more than a thousand crowns for his own education at the university of Pavia.[9]

3

1520-1524

He was registered as a student in the spring of 1520. Pavia was
then a city of scarcely less importance than Milan or Florence.
Here the early kings of Italy were crowned amid elaborate
ceremony; here soldiers of Lombardy defended the city from
behind mighty bastions against the warring factions of the Dark
Ages; churches, palaces, and colleges were built by invaders and
invaded until Pavia became known as "the city of a hundred
towers". In the 8th century the emperor Charlemagne founded
a seat of learning there, and in the 14th, Galeazzo Visconti, son
of the first of the Visconti rulers of Milan, bestowed upon
it the dignity of a university. Galeazzo was a quarrelsome man
who was hated by his Guelph enemies and despised by his
Ghibbeline friends. After one bitter vendetta he and his two
brothers were captured and thrown into jail to await the cruel-
lest of tortures. The two brothers were stripped naked and
flayed with leather thongs until their bodies were reduced to
bleeding pulp, after which swarms of bees were set upon them.
Galeazzo was forced to watch this dreadful sight and left to
think for two days about the similar fate that awaited him. But
his captors were bribed into releasing him and he set about
founding the university as a votive offering for his succour.

At the time of Gerolamo's entry the power of the Visconti
dynasty had waned and that of the Sforzas was in the ascen-
dant. It was a Sforza who had brought Leonardo de Vinci to
Pavia and commissioned him as chief architect of the new
cathedral, which proved almost as great a whirlpool of architec-
tural controversy as had the one in Milan, but which, being
conceived in less gigantic terms, had not suffered the same fate
of excessive ornamentation. And it was Ludovico Sforza, the

seventh Duke of Milan, who had commissioned the extensions
to the University of Pavia which now, in 1520, were approaching completion.[1]

Taking himself on a tour of the city as soon as he is installed
in his tutor's house, Gerolamo notes that the singing in the
cathedral is the finest he has heard. He is pleased that the city is
almost surrounded by water as well as by a "fine great wall of
formidable strength and height". The canals, terraces, and gar-
dens "inspire a tranquil heart even in a body full of turbulent
ills". He finds similar peace in the ancient church of San
Michele "where the stones are worn smooth with the ceremonies
of King-making". Leaving Pavia by the north gate he walks the
five miles to the Certosa di Pavia, the mausoleum of the Visconti built at the end of the 14th century by Gian Galeazzo,
grandson of the Galeazzo who had founded the university. Like
many other Visconti, Gian was vicious and cunning. To his
credit it may be said that he longed to transform Italy from a
land of internecine turmoil into a united nation; but that splendid objective was intended only as a step toward his personal
aggrandisement as despotic ruler of all the provinces and
duchies to be thus unified. He was not, however, to achieve his
ambition in spite of acts of treachery, rapine, and slaughter
against those who opposed him. But he moved a considerable
way toward it by his conquest of Verona, Parma, Como,
Bologna, Pisa, Siena, and Perugia, and kept in his villa at Mar-
ignano* a crown and sceptre ready for his coronation. He was
cheated of further triumphs by the plague and died in 1402,
having ensured that his grandiose life should be marmoreally
recorded in the monastery that he founded.[2] Gerolamo is deeply
impressed by the monastery and reflects that he might well have
found complete peace there if he had carried out his threat,
made during the quarrel with Fazio, to take a monk's cowl.

On the road back to Pavia he falls in with an old man who
acts as agent for a number of corrupt Pavian priests. "He told
me what I knew all too well; that as a youth and a student I
was bound to find many temptations which I should be unable
to resist, but that things could be made easy for me if I wished
to smooth my way with the holy spirit. I supposed he meant the

* Now Melegnano.

sins of lust for which I should be seeking absolution; but the scale of fees he offered bought peace from God for far more odious crimes. Absolution for murder of a parent could be had for a ducat, or for less if not by poisoning. Seven ducats for perjury, twenty for incest with a sister or brother—I cannot recall now all the crimes for which the pardon of Christ could be bought for riches. I told him that such heinous affairs were not for me, whereupon he became threatening and said that I must avail myself of these priests' wares or risk the curses of excommunication. Alarmed, I fled from him, which I could the more easily because of my youthful fleetness and his infirmity, but I heard his raging behind me for a great distance."[3]

This form of religious persecution was beginning by then to die out under the influences of the Reformation; but in an age so much in the shadow of witchcraft the threat of excommunication inspired terrible fear. Witches and wizards could curse, but priests could also: "In the name of the Father, the Son, the Holy Ghost, the blessed Virgin Mary, John the Baptist, Peter and Paul, and all other saints in heaven, do we curse and cut off from our communion him who has thus rebelled against us. May the curse strike him in his house, barn, bed, field, path, city, castle. May he be cursed in battle, accursed in praying, in speaking, in silence, in eating, in drinking, in sleeping. May he be accursed in his taste, hearing, smell, and all his senses. May the curse blast his eyes, head and his body from his crown to the soles of his feet. I conjure you, devil, and all your imps, that you take no rest till you have brought him to eternal shame; till he is destroyed by drowning or hanging, till he is torn to pieces by wild beasts or consumed by fire. Let his children become orphans, his wife a widow. I command you, devil, and all your imps, that even as I now blow out these torches, you do immediately extinguish the light from his eyes. So be it. So be it. Amen. Amen." As the priest ended his curse he would blow out the two wax candles he held in his hands and with that imprimatur the anathema was complete. Men who trembled neither at sword nor fire cowered like slaves before such imprecations on the lips of clergy. Their fellow-men shrank from the wretches thus cursed, and refused communication with them as unclean

and abhorred.[4] The selling of pardons to avoid such excommunication had persisted through most of the Middle Ages and had
enriched the Church and its priests beyond belief. And to the
easy sale of pardons the more corrupt clergy had corruptly
added blackmail—bringing to the confessional poor wretches
who lived lives blameless of any mortal sins, but from whom
sins and money for absolution had to be extorted. In this practice the priests put themselves on a par with modern gangsters
who sell "protection" to the innocent. Gerolamo was wise to be
alarmed and to flee. He reports no further trouble from corrupt
clerics; and indeed by 1520 the blatant sale of absolutions for
any crime in the calendar had been temporarily diminished by
the influential humanism of Erasmus and the reforming zeal of
Martin Luther.

Gerolamo's tutor at Pavia was a scholar named Giovanni Targio. He directed the young man's studies toward the attainment
of a Bachelor of Arts degree, which would be necessary before
he could specialize in medicine. He also noted Gerolamo's
achievements and moral and physical defects. "He was quick
always to grasp the tenets of his interests. Laconic and witty in
speech, he gave offence too often for his life to be free of
enemies. He turned conversation from him by his concern for
his health, on which he would dissemble for hours while companions dwindled. He could be merry for an hour and glum for
a day. He contrived his own way of studying, which was soli-
tary and seldom done in the hall with other students. Each
morning he spent in the library, then walked a little outside the
town walls in the shade before he dined frugally in his own
room, cooking what he needed and drawing the wine from a
butt beside his bed. After that he would find companionship for
an hour, but only where there would be music—which, if it
were nowhere to be found among friends he would seek in the
churches. Thus refreshed, he would leave the city gates again
and find small deserted streams among the woods and groves
where he could sit fishing, his ink-horn and paper beside him for
his thoughts to be freed, until at sunset he would return to the
town for drinking and gambling in the taverns and walking late
in the streets, disguised and with sword drawn, in peril of arrest

for contravening the law but determined to live some fantasy life of his own connected with the dreadful dreams from which he suffered and which were incensed by his reading of the *Malleus Maleficarum.** In these dreams processions of faceless figures, seemingly built of rings of mail, passed before him and always were followed by a cock with red wings that screamed in a terrible voice and uttered human words that held threats that dissolved in waking memory, only leaving him exhausted with fear and in a trembling sweat."[5]

It is not surprising that the celebrated work on witchcraft should have sent startling fantasies through a mind so introverted as Gerolamo's. The current of demonology had by the 15th century become so electric in its effect that inquisitors working under the auspices of the Church could command the most awful deaths on those suspected of working with the Devil. That the Church itself was rotten with moral corruption was of no account—or, rather, of a different account, an account to be settled by the Erasmuses and Luthers of the approaching Reformation. The inquisitors gathered evidence against all women supposed to be in league with the Devil and thereby able to curse, to cause pain and impotence and disfigurement, to render the fields useless and the crops destroyed by pestilence. Inquisitorial methods were supposed to be just and to bring into force, in the early stages of the sentence "only the mildest forms of torture to encourage confession". But the mildest forms of torture were whipping, the thumbscrew, and stretching on the rack or ladder. These were often believed by the judges to be useless against the powers of those invested with devils and were therefore ignored "so that time should not be wasted in the despatch or recantment of God's enemies". The slow dismemberment of the toes and fingers, the slow burning over fires of green wood; the tearing off of the eyelids and nipples with iron pincers, while the body, weighted with iron weights, was hoisted into the air by the strappado and jerked up and down like a puppet on a string and the entrails leaked out through slashes in the belly as the mutilated but still living witch hung bleeding and broken above the inquisitors—these were some of the more advanced

* The work on witchcraft by Sprenger and Kramer, which had been published in 1486 and was in wide circulation in Europe.

forms of torture prescribed in the *Malleus* as witches' punishment, and were nightmares in themselves. It may well have been with some notion of enfeebling their grip upon his dreams that Gerolamo walked "late in the streets, disguised . . . determined to live some fantasy life of his own". In a credulous age, he would have been acting quite normally in stalking the phantoms of disquiet with sword and mask.

But though Gerolamo grumbles ceaselessly of bodily ailments, he has little to say of his mental fantasies. And for a good reason : the way to the exploration of the mind's darker areas had not yet been pointed out by Descartes, who belongs to the succeeding century. The mind was to be used for the study of things outside itself. And during his first academic year Gerolamo studied intensively. His advancement was so fast that Targio allowed him occasionally to teach Euclid, while he took part many times in the public debates. By the time he was twenty-one he was also appointed as a teacher of dialectics and philosophy. Throughout that time he was writing treatise after treatise on mathematics, geometry, and music. And as preparation for his medical studies he prepared a thesis *On The Differing Opinions of Physicians*. Between the academic sessions he sometimes returned to Milan, sometimes stayed in residence with Targio.[6] Gambling, music, and fencing were his only recreations, and gambling began to take an ever larger part in his daily life, for it had now become the subject of a special mathematical study that was to be called *Liber de Ludo Aleae—The Book on Games of Chance*. For this, he returned to the formulae he had worked out during the time he had been winning the money that was supporting him at Pavia.

Gerolamo was never a compulsive gambler. Unlike such addicts, he had no hidden desire to lose, to find orgasmic relief, compensation for some deep-centred frustration, in contemplating the successive stages of financial ruination. From a primary concern with winning enough money to take him to the university, his interest had developed into a scientific one. He did not investigate what today we should call "systems", for all systems must be founded on laws defining the probability of chances. It was those laws that he was able to set forth in *Liber de Ludo Aleae*.

In truth, the work that in due course was to bring Gerolamo some fame is of muddled composition. He frequently worked out a solution to a problem, later discovered that he was in error, and confusingly left both the wrong and the right answers without any indication of the links between them. He mixed moral, practical, historical, and mathematical aspects of gambling indiscriminately, and often failed to clarify his meaning. But he did not fail to express with perfect clarity the first Law of Probability. He began his cogitations logically enough by considering that a die has six sides and that in a single cast of the die, since only chance is involved, any one of the sides is as likely to fall uppermost as any other. "There are six equally likely cases", he wrote, and expressed it arithmetically with the fraction $\frac{1}{6}$. Thus, for determining the probability of an event that is governed by pure chance, as in a game of dice, the formula to be observed is $p = f/c$, p being the probability, c the total number of possible cases, and f the total number of favourable cases. Applied to the tossing of a coin, the fraction would be $\frac{1}{2}$, since there are two sides to the coin and one chance in a single toss that either side will fall uppermost. "The probability of an event," he continued, "is the number of cases favourable to that event compared with the total number of possible cases, so long as all the possible cases are equally likely to happen." He then went on to calculate the probabilities with two or three dice, and arrived at formulae that would show the player precisely what were the odds against his throwing any particular number with two or three dice—knowledge that would enable him to decide the amount of his stake, or whether, indeed, he should place a stake at all. Then Gerolamo crystallized the entire orbit of chance in the words, "Events may be of three kinds : the impossible (as it might be the throwing of a 7 with a single die), the certain (as the certainty that one side of a thrown die must fall uppermost), and the probable (as it might be that a 6 should fall uppermost at the first throw of the die). If the impossible is set down as 0 and the certain as 1, then all the degrees of probability in between the extremes may be calculated in fractions".[7] Nowadays, it all seems very obvious and of small account. Few experienced gamblers putting their stake on a number in roulette, a throw in craps, or a card in *chemin de fer* are unaware of the odds against them and the odds in their favour at any particular stage of the game; but even fewer know, and fewer still care, that it was Gerolamo Cardano who plucked out of the arithmetical mysteries of the early 16th century the equations that they bring, as unthinkingly as they arrive at the sum of one plus one, to their support.

Liber de Ludo Aleae was not published for some years; but Gerolamo's labours on it had successful results at the gaming tables. "Though I lost as often as I won, I was, by benefit of my calculations, rarely a loser of great sums; but by wily reckoning, when it came my fortune to win, then the sums I won were of greater size, so that my nightly turns at the tables were of considerable resource to me." In a letter written about this time to a fellow student, Ottaviano Scoto, he eulogizes the happiness of his life at Pavia. Writing from Milan, where he is staying between sessions of the academic year, he says that, fond though he is of his parents, he finds that detachment from them and his aunt is very welcome. His studies are going well; his health, "though far from any degree of perfection" is at the moment troubling him less. Targio is pleased with him and there is every chance that he will shortly achieve his Baccalaureat and take up his further studies in medicine. "I look forward to seeing you, my good friend, on my return to Pavia, and to renewing my tranquil days in learning".[8] He was not, however, to return to Pavia to continue his tranquil life. War and plague were to intervene.

4

1525

King Louis XII was succeeded on the throne of France by his son-in-law, Francis I. The struggle for the domination of Europe was now concentrated in the rivalry between Francis and Charles, the Habsburg prince who was to become the Emperor Charles V. Francis, aged twenty-one, succeeded on 1 January 1515, and four days later Charles, a boy of fifteen, was declared of age and invested with the monarchy of Spain and the Netherlands. Francis's first step toward the hegemony of Europe was to acquire the Duchy of Milan, which he did bloodlessly, for Maximilian Sforza, the reigning duke, surrendered to him without opposition and abdicated immediately. Francis installed a French governor in the city and for six years ruled it by proxy until, in 1521, Charles forced out the occupying French troops and installed his own. They remained there for three years but in their turn were forced by a new epidemic of plague to relinquish their merciless grip on the city. In that year, 1524, fifty thousand people were stricken. Their hideously ravaged bodies were pitchforked daily into death-carts and dragged to the piazza before the cathedral, where they were posthumously given the last rites of the Church and burnt. Month after month a great pall of smoke hung over the city. Those occupying troops who escaped death marched out and camped in the surrounding countryside. But gradually it became impossible to get supplies to them and eventually they dispersed and sought other ducal factions that would hire them as mercenaries. As the population dwindled in the great funeral pyre Francis saw his chance to repossess the Duchy. He waited till the plague had spent itself, then marched into the city with a great army of

French and Swiss troops. There he learnt that some four thousand of Charles's German and Spanish troops had escaped to
Pavia, where they had taken possession of the castle, which they
were defending with sixteen pieces of artillery. Francis immediately detached a body of his own men and led them in an attack
on the castle. He was bloodily repulsed and retreated hurriedly
to the edge of the huge park that surrounded the castle. Since
Francis had four times the number of defensive guns that were
ranged behind the ramparts of the castle, and was amply sup-
plied with ammunition and stores, he saw no difficulty in besieg-
ing the place. It was simply a matter of time and patience. For
three months he persisted in his efforts. But meanwhile Charles's
famous General, Georg von Frundsberg, had assembled an
immense band of German mercenaries and was approaching
Pavia from the north-east, skirting Milan under cover of darkness and arriving at the north wall of the park with no warning
of their approach having reached Francis's ears. For three weeks
there were skirmishes both inside and outside the park walls.
Then von Frundsberg breached the wall with artillery and bat-
tering rams and the tremendous climactic battle was fought
within the great park. It ended with the complete rout of the
French, "All the chivalry of France, followed by the panic-
stricken Swiss, fleeing in terror before the belching artillery of
their assailants."[1] Francis had his horse killed beneath him and
was trampled on by his own cavalry. In that piteous state, his
gorgeous robes stained with blood and mud, his silver tunic
slashed by lances, his gold chain of St Michael and his helmet
plume and sword belt wrenched off him by the soldiery, he
surrendered to Charles's viceroy, Lannoy. "Lannoy, deeply
moved by the humiliation of the king, knelt and kissed his hand,
and received, kneeling, the sword that Francis offered him,
offering him in turn his own. Then other commanders in
Charles's forces came and did reverence to the fallen monarch".[2] Thus ended the battle of Pavia.

During those ten years from 1515 to 1525 Gerolamo's life, as
I have shown, was tranquil and orderly. Whether Milan was
occupied by French or Imperialist troops made little difference
to the lives of the people—certainly not to a student, morose in
disposition, who was concerned rather with science and the

humanities than with politics. Writing of his years at Pavia he makes no reference to the decimating outbreak of plague in 1524, for the disease was a commonplace; and of his inability to return to the university he remarks only, "War closed the academy that year, and when it was over there was no money to reorganize its activities". The battle that ended in the triumph of Charles's forces and revealed to him the prospect of a boundless empire—which he all but achieved before, exhausted by gluttony and other physical excesses, he abdicated in 1556—meant little to Gerolamo. Splendour, conquest, military affairs, were outside his consideration. He was concerned only to achieve his doctorate in medicine. With the Baccalaureat to his credit he had no difficulty in taking up his studies again, this time at the university of Padua, which was to Venice as Pavia was to Milan. Its charter had been granted in 1238, and medicine and the arts were given equal prominence with civil and canon law—except in the matter of the teachers' stipends, which, for those who taught jurisprudence, were twenty times as great. "But since I was being taught and not teaching, this was reflected only in the humour of those who taught me, and I minded it not".[3]

He had scarcely started his term at the university when he was recalled to Milan because Fazio was dying. The old man was eighty and there was nothing to be done for him. His mind was still bright and he lay peacefully, between the snoozes of senility, listening to Gerolamo and a student colleague of his answering his many questions about life at Padua. Like all old men, he was interested in the changes that had taken place since his own student days, and shook his head in dismay when Gerolamo told him that because of the turmoil caused by wars no Rector had been appointed for some years and that he himself was being considered for this important office of administrative head of the university. Understandably, Fazio could not credit that such a retrograde step should be taken as to consider appointing a young man in his early twenties, newly graduated from another university and lacking both the social and financial qualifications required for the post. It seems most likely that Gerolamo, perhaps urged by Chiara, was trying to lighten his father's last days with gratifying pride. The university records reveal nothing whatever about the appointment of Gerolamo as Rector, nor that he was ever considered for election. On the contrary, they mention specifically that there was an interregnum in the Rectorship between 1515 and 1528. In spite of that, however, Gerolamo refers several times in his many autobiographical writings to the period of his Rectorship, and gloomily adds that it was "disastrous" because of the financial obligations involved. As indeed it would have been. Whether or not he ever wore the robes of purple and gold and the cross of Saint Mark, and assumed the Rectorial functions, must remain a mystery. But it is no mystery that Fazio died on 28 October 1525, possibly still puzzling over the depths to which a great university could sink by considering as its administrator an ill-conceived youth with neither money nor wisdom.

Gerolamo returned to Padua in time for the opening of the academic year on All Saints'-day, Fazio having been speedily buried at the church of Saint Mark, Milan. His father's death left him in great distress, and it was only because he could immerse himself in his studies immediately that he was able to stop brooding on it. His tutor was Matthew Curtius, who was professor of medicine at Padua, and a doctor of considerable distinction in his day. He had written on venesection in pleurisy and was the editor of the standard textbook of anatomy. He was a man of fifty and an extremely able teacher. "So clear was his instruction," says Cardano, "that within a year I was able to present myself to the faculty". Since the normal course of instruction was for nine terms, Curtius's teaching must have been brilliant indeed; but Gerolamo's capacity for learning equalled it. Teacher and student were in fact of matched talents, and no doubt both took pleasure in the challenge of an application for examination after only three terms.

In those days the granting of a degree in medicine depended as much on social qualification as upon proof of ability in healing. Admission to the faculty resembled passage through the committee of some exclusive club. Technical qualification was to be proved by public debate in the hall of the university. The candidate there had to present two theses of his own and argue the merits and demerits of two others presented by his opponents. That part of the examination Gerolamo passed with honours. He confounded his opponents by demolishing all their traps and proved invincible in arguing his own theses. He was accorded an ovation and together with his sponsors withdrew from the hall while a ballot was taken. "Here," he records, "I was disappointed of success. No doubt the disgrace attaching to my bastardy, the odium of my attendance so frequently in places where dice and cards were the idols, and my rudeness in dispute, were more than these sages of the faculty could digest. Forty-seven were against my admission and nine in my favour. I was angry and persuaded my presentors to plead my cause in another election. This time there were more for me, but again more than half rejected me. But Francisco Buonafede* urged upon the faculty yet another election, and at last I was accepted, by an exact reversal of the first ballot, there being now forty-seven in my favour and nine who rejected me. So I came at last to my laureat, being twenty-five years in age and my life more than past the meridian and now in decline—as I then believed, for had not my astrologers said that my birth was ill-favoured by the stars and that death would overtake me before I had forty-five years, and that premonitions of my death would be many and fateful? As so they were."[4]

These "premonitions" can be included with his dreams, nightmares, and daytime fantasies, as being the object of a concern that was commoner in days when the mind was an even vaster mystery than it is today. That Gerolamo was not fey in the sense of being prophetically apprehensive of his own death is proved by the fact that he long outlived the urgent premonitions that he notes with boring frequency. One such will be sufficient example. "Twice in a morning, once while I still lay abed and again when I was dressing, I heard several sharp raps as with a hammer on the wall of the room where I lodged. Yet the chamber beyond that wall was completely empty, so what could those knockings mean but the peremptory summons, or warning, of death? In this case it was the death of my father's old friend, Galeazzo Rosso, who, I learned, died within the hour encompassed by the knocking. But I was not to be comforted by any

* Professor of practical medicine at Padua and one of Gerolamo's sponsors.

respite. In this or some similar manner, I knew, would come the
summons for me."[5] He writes of this and scores of similar "premonitions", nearly half a century later, and it is far from clear
whether he intends to disparage himself for his foolish fancies or
whether he still clings to the belief that death will make its
fateful announcement. But certainly he did not shed his morbi-
dity.

On the very day of the ceremony of his installation he is
stricken with "stabbing pains in the limbs and a flux in the
head". He lists, in four pages, every bodily defect he finds that
morning. A minute examination of his flesh reveals bruises,
abrasions, scars, tender spots, infections. He can eat nothing,
and a little wine turns his stomach "into a tempest". He sends
his servant for goat's milk and wonders whether he will ever be
able to endure the rigours of the day. But all seems to have
passed off well. He presented himself to the bishop for examination in loyalty and orthodoxy in the christian faith, and to the
priest for confession and communion; then in the hall of the
university he was offered by the senior professors in succession
the symbols of his laureation. These were an open book, symbo-
lizing all that was known to him and that he might teach; a
closed book, for all that had yet to learn; the biretta that consecrated him as a priest of science; the ring that espoused him to
medicine; and the kiss of brotherhood given him by all his
mentors as they filed before him and made obeisance to their
new colleague. The entire assembly then moved in procession to
the Basilica of Saint Antonio, where the final ceremonial of his
enthronement took place. This ceremonial was of crowning sig-
nificance. The prior of the basilica, in the habit of a Franciscan,
sat upon a plain chair at one end of the refectory and at his
right hand was a second chair, equally plain. At the other end
of the refectory were gathered the preceptors of the university,
Gerolamo and his sponsors on a separate bench before them. At
the proper moment the court usher tapped his staff twice upon
the ground and Gerolamo, carrying his biretta, was led by his
sponsors across the refectory to the prior. Genuflections to the
prior were made, a mime of the presentation was gone through,
and the prior gestured to Gerolamo to seat himself upon the

empty chair at his side. The sponsors bowed again and withdrew and the usher spoke the only words used throughout the ceremony : "Gerolamo Cardano, laureate in medicine, you are now by your learning qualified to sit among the princes of the earth. Go, and heal those who need you."

In that way Gerolamo became Doctor Cardano.

5

1525–1531

The very next day he travelled to Milan on horseback. It was a long and unpleasant journey made for the most part in pouring rain and thunderstorms. He was accompanied by his servant Tomasini, a simple-minded fellow who more than once left behind in the inns where they lodged various pieces of Cardano's baggage, necessitating frequent retracings of ground already covered. These delays and the appalling conditions of the roads that circumnavigated the foothills of the Alps elongated the distance to close on two hundred miles and the time to five days. By the time they reached Milan the fledgling doctor had become so depressed by his broodings that he thought morbidly of taking a draught "that would vanquish all ills for ever, and life with them".[1] The main subject of his gloomy introversion during the journey seems to have been his sexual impotence. Whether he was so sure of this further defect in himself because he had failed to sire any children upon paramours, or whether he was simply unable to achieve erection or orgasm, is not clear. The latter seems by far the more probable, since there is very little evidence of his sexual association with female partners in his student days. There is, however, a strong suggestion that he was a voyeur* and a frequent masturbator. It is possible that the mental guilt associated with these practices had the psychological effect of impotence. But his youthful days were so ridden with hypochondria that it is difficult to believe that he suffered from more than a tiny proportion of the ills he debited himself with. That they were very real to the contortions of his gloomy self-study, however, is certain.

---

* His *voyeurism* was directed at obscene drawings, paintings and sculptures rather than at persons engaged in sexual congress.

And he says in a letter to Francisco Buonafede, sent soon after he arrived in Milan, that his impotence is the greatest of his troubles.

"I maintain that this misfortune is to me the worst of evils. Compared with it, neither the harsh servitude under my father, nor unkindness, nor the troubles of litigation, nor the wrongs done me by my fellow townsmen, nor the scorn of my fellow physicians, nor the ill things spoken against me nor all the measureless mass of possible evil, could have brought me to such despair, and distaste of all pleasure, and lasting sorrow. I bitterly weep this misery, that I must needs be a laughing-stock, that marriage must be denied me, and that I must ever live in solitude. You ask for the cause of this misfortune, a matter which I am quite unable to explain. But because of it, and because I dread that men shall know how grave is the ill afflicting me, I shun the society of women; and on account of this habit, followed only to shun miserable public scandal, I bring upon myself the very scandal I desire to avoid, together with the suspicion of still more nefarious practices. In sooth it seems that there is no further calamity for me to endure."

Such dismal outpourings, whether made in letter or conversation, were unlikely to make him popular; and it is worth noting that most of the friends he made while a student at Pavia drifted away from him as he became more concerned with his ills, real or imagined, and more wearisome in his determination to retell his dreams and apprehensions. Possibly the intensive studies for his doctorate had increased his hypochondria. But he certainly set out for Milan full of high hopes of establishing a practice there. "He bade me farewell in great wit," his other sponsor, Matthew Curtius, records; "and assured me that soon we should be meeting at the College [of Physicians in Milan]." In that, however, both doctors were to be disappointed. Cardano went at once to see his mother, and from her to interview the Principal of the College. He carried letters of introduction from the faculty at Padua and wore his biretta and ring. But the College would have none of him. Some ill-wisher recalled the matter of his bastardy and pointed out that the statutes of the College required all who applied for membership to be "born within the degree of holy marriage". Which was true, and perhaps as good an excuse as any for scorning his application; but the rule had been disregarded many times before and could have been on this occasion too if the authorities so wished. It seems far more likely that they rejected the new doctor's application because he was known to be aggressive in argument, boringly self-pitying, and critical of established medical practice Had he not written a paper, barbed with cynical comment, *On The Differing Opinions of Physicians*? If he could write such fomenting criticism while still a student, what might he not do in the fuller authority of his qualification? The sages of the College were doubtless more fearful of his perspicacity than they were disapproving of his bastardy. A bright new intellect could too easily unravel the cocoon of traditional beliefs that were handed down from generation to generation like comfortable suits of clothes whose increasing thinness they preferred to ignore. At all events, they refused him membership of the College; and by doing so barred him from practice in Milan. "So they have turned me away from the wealth of my true city." he told Chiara, "and spurned the help I could give the sick." This reaction was uncharacteristically mercenary and arrogant. Cardano had little regard for wealth in excess of necessity, and was by nature too self-critical to believe in his as yet unproven powers as a healer. But it was an understandable reaction all the same. He wished to express lofty disregard for the College's rejection, though the impression must have been one of self-pitying sulks. In due course, he would wreak a more effective, and more malicious, revenge.

He remained in Milan for some months, well aware of the loss of dignity that would result from a scuttling away from the city like a whipped dog. There was in any case much tiresome business for him to attend to. Fazio's death had involved him in litigation over his inheritance, and legal wrangles were to persist for years. The small amount of property Fazio left was scarcely worth the trouble, but principle was at stake and Gerolamo fought for that rather than for the material advantage of a few rents, a little jewellery, and a collection of dusty legal and medical tomes. He must have often recalled wryly his childhood opinion that litigation was "the pursuit of ends through the passages of a maze".

Those other ends, the setting up of a practice and continued study in medicine, having been denied him in Milan, he went, on the advice of Francisco Buonafede, to Sacco, a small town a few miles from Padua. "There is no physician established there," Buonafede wrote; "yet the demands are considerable. I am at all times making use of your name as one who will serve the people well." He may well have done that, for he had a warm heart and a great admiration for his pupil. But so far as business was concerned the demand for a doctor's services seem to have vanished as soon as Cardano arrived—if, indeed, that demand was not measured too optimistically by Buonafede. In anticipation of earning a proper living Cardano bought a small house at Sacco, using such savings as he had been able to accumulate from gambling and tutorial fees. He moved to it on his birthday, 24 September 1526, and waited for patients. Few patients called for him in spite of the fact that there was a fair amount of sickness in the town. The people preferred the services of sorcerers and priests, whose treatments were more dramatic and less concerned with physical self-discipline. He was, however, welcomed in the town as a distinguished man of letters and treated with great respect. The mayor presented him to the populace in the town hall; the captain of the garrison, Altobello Bandarini, who had in his charge three companies of Venetian state troops, ordered that Cardano should be given the honours due to a field officer each time he passed a sentry; and the many minor nobles of Venice who administered the town asked him into their homes for music and conversation. Cardano fills many pages describing the *conversazione* occasions at which he was a guest. His descriptions of some of the quaint parlour games the company amused themselves with are somewhat acid. "Throughout a single evening we played the game of Solitude, in which first a King or Queen is elected by lot and then severally the company must decide what manner of solitude they would choose if forced to it by the unrequited love of a lady. As one might say, 'I would withdraw to Mount Olympus, where I shall prove whether the proverb be true, "Out of sight, out of mind" '; and another, 'I shall go to the solitude of a desert that in humbling myself thus I shall be exalted in heaven'; and another, 'I shall devote myself to God in a holy

monastery'. It was a great fidget to me that I who could have
told them so much of solitude could not do so in so pithy a
form, with an epigram or proverb, for my tale would have been
longer and bitterer and I should have seemed impolite in such
delicate company." But if he is not pleased with the conversation and the supper—which, he says, is "too full of pastry and
viands filled with spice"—he is pleased when the musicians with
lutes and lyres fill the gallery above the dining hall "and make
sounds more worthy of human ears that all the idle chatter of
supper time".

If his residence in Sacco did little else for him, it accomplished two things: it taught him, anyway in small measure, to
accommodate his unruly tongue to the demands of a society in
which he was no longer a mere youth whose ill-bred outbursts
could be scorned, but a man of position whose irritability could
be attributed to the crankiness of scholarship. It also brought
him a wife—in circumstances that made him tremble with
apprehension, "they were so strange and luminary". Luminary
indeed. One night a comet appeared directly over the town
causing Cardano's head to be "filled with troubled lightnings"
as to what it might portend. Since he had some knowledge of
astronomy he is surprisingly unscientific in leaping immediately
to the superstitious conclusion that the comet was a fateful sign
for him and him alone; but so he was. "I was alone, sitting on a
tombstone when the streak of golden stars appeared. I was
abroad without hindrance since the captain had given orders
that I was frequently about at night because of my sleeplessness,
and the soldiers knew my route. I stretched at once in fright
upon the stone, all the equations that had been my consideration gone from my head, and a great fear filling it instead. The
town was asleep, and I took myself home at great speed." The
morning might have brought him to the conclusion that comets
could presage benign as well as harmful events; but the night
turned out to be fuller still of dramatic incident. He had no
sooner put himself to bed and fallen into a troubled sleep when
he had a dream. "I seemed to find myself in a pleasant garden,
beautiful exceedingly, filled with flowers and soft fruits the like
of which were amazing. Even the air was of a particular beauty.
So lovely was it that no painter nor our poet Pulci, nor any

imagination of man could have figured the like. I was standing
in the forecourt of this garden, the door being open, and there
was another door on the opposite side. Of a sudden that other
door opened and in its frame stood a woman, a most beautiful
woman. I embraced and kissed her, and in the very act of
kissing her the door was closed and the garden vanished and we
were in total darkness, she and I, and I was full of nameless
fears so that I awoke suddenly, sweating and troubled." He had
not long been awake when he heard sounds of great alarm in
the street below. Fire had broken out somewhere and people
were hurrying to the scene. Cardano of course had to join them,
his mind and heart even fuller now of the forebodings that had
been started by the comet. The house on fire, he soon learnt,
was that in which lived the captain of the garrison, Bandarini.
Mercifully, the captain and his family were staying in Padua at
the time, but the house was gutted. That resulted in a move for
the Bandarinis when they returned, and it chanced that they
moved into the house that adjoined Cardano's. There were, he
now learnt, four daughters and four sons in the family; and he
is exasperated by the arrival next door of a "family of so great a
size that there can scarcely be any peace from their comings and
goings". However, a few days later he encountered one of the
daughters as she emerged from the house; and at once he was
put into another great fever of emotion; for there before him
was the girl of his dream.

To us of the latter part of the 20th century, steeped as we
are in the explanation of dreams imparted by such analysts
as Freud and Dunne, there is nothing specially remarkable in
Cardano's experience. But to him, living in an age afflicted by
superstition and the terrors of the inexplicable, and having a
character that continually wavered between mental brilliance
and emotional wretchedness, there must have been great turbu-
lence of spirit. He saw signs in everything. A dog howls and he
is certain that this is a portent of death for "my new-found love
Lucia Bandarini"; a few ravens gather on the roof and begin
croaking and this will mean a grave illness for himself; his
servant breaks up a faggot and sparks fly out of it, "which can
mean nothing but another visitation of war and pestilence". For
days he broods, filled with querulous self-questioning. "What is

this girl to me? If I, poor wretch that I am, take to wife a girl dowered with naught, except a crowd of brothers and sisters, it will be all over with me; for I can hardly keep myself as it is. If I should attempt to carry her off, or to have my will of her by stealth, there will surely be some tale-bearers to witness; and her father, being a fellow-townsman and a soldier to boot, would not sit down lightly under such an injury. In this case or that it is hard to say what course I should follow, for if this affair should come to the issue I most desire, I must needs fly the place.

"Those were the thoughts, and others like them, that from the hour of our meeting possessed my brain, which was only too ready to harbour them, and I felt it would be better to die than to live on in such perplexity. Thenceforth I was as one burnt up with passion, and I understood what meaning I might gather from the reading of my dream, for I was suddenly freed from the chain of impotence that had held me back from marriage."

Somewhat disingenuously, he goes on to say that every night now his bed is "rocked with great tremblings and divers noises which can only be the work of demons adding to my discomfiture". If he could believe that he could believe anything. Whatever he believed, he was unable to resist further the blandishments of the dreamy Lucia; and he married her on 14 November 1531.

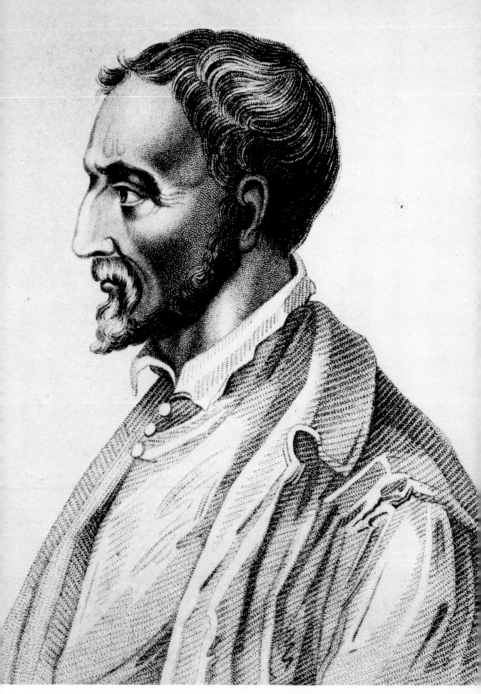

Gerolamo Cardano, 1501–76

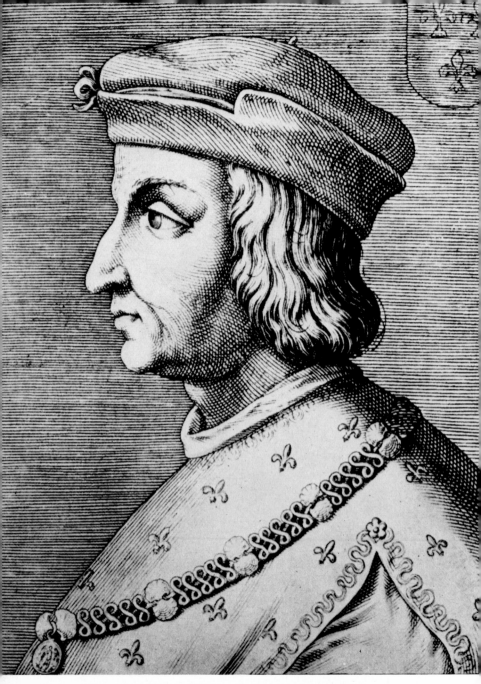

Louis XII, King of France during Cardano's childhood

6

1532–1534

Five years have elapsed since Cardano came to Sacco. He is thirty years old and has great prestige as a citizen but no renown as a doctor. He is still filled with bitter resentment against the College of Physicians in Milan for denying him his right to practice in the great city. That resentment he keeps muffled inside him for fear that, if he reveals it, people will take the view that there is no smoke without fire and that he is guilty as well as malicious.

So far as his father-in-law is concerned he has made a great conquest. Bandarini, a fat and genial fellow with a fat purse to match, has the highest regard and affection for Cardano. Delighted by the match Lucia has made, he generously offers to support them in proper style for so long as they care to remain in Sacco. Immediately, Cardano's independence of spirit crustily asserts itself and he turns the offer down. Lucia is now his responsibility, he says with worthy fervour, and he will support her "in however poor a hovel".[1] They will leave Sacco at once, return to Milan, and set up house in the face of all challenges. Bandarini is at first distressed by such talk, then angered. His plans for his cherished daughter do not include penniless residence in a hovel or ignominy cast upon her by a clique of Milanese snobs. His distress and anger are matched by Cardano's obstinacy. Nothing will serve but complete severance from his father-in-law's support. Lucia, dutiful to both father and husband, is grieved that she should be at the centre of so much contention. There are arguments galore. Bandarini's geniality vanishes behind a military determination to secure his objective. Cardano lets fly with the weapons of scorn and sarcasm. The ambiance becomes strongly redolent of that prevail-

3—DC * *

ing in the Cardano household in the days of Gerolamo's childhood and youth. But, surprisingly, Bandarini suddenly gives way—perhaps with the subtlety of a strategist who withdraws from a minor battle so that he may later trap the enemy in a major one. He consents, with his blessing, to the departure of the newly married couple to Milan and tells them they must follow whatever way of life they choose so long as filial devotion is not threatened. But whatever the subtlety behind his intention in this sudden *volte face*, we can never discover it, for he died less than a year later—possibly of poison administered by his eldest son, who had designs on his wealth.

When Cardano moved to Milan in February 1532, Lucia was pregnant. But he took with him children of his mind as well as of his flesh. His five years in Sacco, lacking in his medical practice though they were, had borne fruit in the form of a number of manuscripts. Among them was the *Book on Games of Chance,* which he had revised (and was to revise many times again). There was also a treatise on chiromancy. This means of prophesying the events of a life from the study of the hands was, with astrology, geomancy, and other methods of divination, widely popular in those days. "The hand," he wrote in the preface to the treatise, "is the instrument of the body, as the tongue is of the mind." The treatise itself is in much the same unoriginal strain, a mere digest of all that had been written before, and to which, indeed, very little has been added since. The parts of the hand are named—carpus, thenar, hypothenar, stethos—and the fingers are allotted their "controlling" planets—Mars to the thumb, Jove to the index finger, Saturn to the third, the Sun to the fourth, and Venus to the fifth; and there are many interpretations of life-, head-, and heart-lines, and readings of the configuration of the white spots on the fingernails. It is clear that Cardano puts a very high value on divination by palmistry (to give it its modern name). It may seem strange for a man with a scientific mind to be so interested in such occult and superstitious matters as divination, amulets, dreams, spirit manifestations, and witchcraft; but such beliefs were the heritage of the period—and, indeed, many of them still prevail in the 20th century, for mercifully it is not yet within the scope of human knowledge to rationalize everything. In any case, yesterday's explorations of the supernatural often led to the establishment of today's sciences. They did so in the case of two more of the manuscripts Cardano took with him to Milan. These were treatises on divination from the study of handwriting and from the study of the lines and blemishes on the human face. Both graphology and metoposcopy have become recognized sciences for the study of character if not of fortune. And if Cardano did not "invent" them he at least, in those treatises, advanced them to the stage at which they could be seen to have scientific justification.

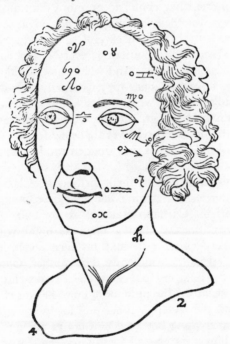

Cardano's studies in metoposcopy emphasized the importance of the positions of facial warts

The visit to Milan was a disaster. Lucia miscarried a month later and the treatises too proved abortive, for no one would publish them. And though in five years Cardano had acquired a civic if not a medical reputation in Sacco, and that reputation was eulogized in letters of introduction, the College of Physicians showed no change of heart toward him. His admission was still forbidden and he was treated with lofty disdain by the entire hierarchy, from the President downward. Those gentlemen doctors, all exquisitely dressed and accoutred, had flourishing practices nurtured by the élite of the city, whom they attended with grave bedside demeanour, consulting among themselves in the sick-rooms of each wealthy patron, as if the recovery of a state official or a guild merchant from a bout of indigestion might influence the future of Europe. When faced with plague, typhus, or enteric, they could do no more than anyone else—in fact rather less, for their learning had not advanced since their student days. But they were careful to introduce "new" prophylactics, possets, and poultices at every deathbed to give the effect of esoteric knowledge. And when those antidotes failed, as fail they were bound to, since they were only old vinegar-soaked kerchiefs, mulled herbal wine, and sulphur plasters masquerading under different names, the physicians conferred again and reported to the bereaved relatives that new forms of the diseases had broken out. After that they divided the fees equably among themselves, attended requiems for the souls of the departed, and contributed handsomely to their memorials. Clearly it was in their own interests that their circle should remain closed.

All the patients Cardano managed to treat in Milan he had to treat surreptitiously, visiting them at night with his cloak wrapped closely about him and his face concealed within a cowl. He raged at such indignity. His mother, Chiara, tried to soothe him by pointing out that he was proving himself an excellent physician by the number of cures he was effecting. That was true. And the fact that they were lowly and often criminal people he was treating bothered him not at all; nor did the lack of fees. His bitterness was all for the secrecy, for the exclusions from discussion with his rightful colleagues, for his inability to meet the great need for more doctors in the city—a need which Louis XII had noted on the very day, twenty-three years before, when the child Gerolamo had determined on his career. The irony was like a wound that would not heal. He sought relief for it by planning a treatise on fate, opening it with an exposition of his own life up to that present, a new examination of his horoscope in conjunction with astrological observations, and contemplation of the machinations of fortune. "In those days I was sickened so to the heart that I would visit diviners and wizards so that some solution might be found to my manifold troubles. Many of them advised me, as it might be that on certain days I should drink only from cups that had contained ochre, that on other certain days I should walk only on the left side of the arcades and shield myself from the moon's rays, or that on waking I should sneeze three times and knock on wood. Though I was at great pains to follow these advices they availed me nothing. And of all the observations I made of the night sky and of the conjunctions of the stars at my own birth, none offered me hope for many months, for the planets crossed in their courses and made a mockery of my life. And peer into the multitude of lines on my hand though I might, and scatter the grains* in boundless number, yet there was no hope for me there in Milan. I was forced to the dice again so that I could support my wife; and here my knowledge defeated fortune and we were able to buy food and live, though our lodgings were desolate, the while I worked far into the night on my book explaining Fate."[3]

His explanations of the workings of fate were limited to a gloomy accumulation of his family misfortunes. He could point to his father's early efforts to overcome the resentment shown by the jurisconsults of Milan and compare them with his own fight against the prejudices of the doctors, drawing the conclusion that "a choler in the blood of all Cardanos makes us subject to the contempt of our inferiors". He could find similar fateful explanations for Chiara's licentiousness, Lucia's miscarriage, and the litigation over Fazio's patrimony. "Events frequently happen contrary to human wishes, and such disappointments must be borne with equanimity".[4] Indeed, that is Christian ethic. But while Cardano was writing with such humility about his lot in life, he was displaying to those around him a very different attitude. The social graces he had acquired for the benefit of the

---

* In geomancy, a small container of sand is scattered over a paper chart ruled off into squares, and the resulting configuration of grains "read", rather as tea leaves are interpreted to divine the future.

sophisticated company in Sacco now fell from him. He was irascible at home, so that Lucia was sorely tried by his temper as well as by poverty; he vented his spleen against the College of Physicians in a loud voice as he roamed about the city, giving the impression of an unbalanced mind; in company in the taverns where he gambled he swore unwisely malicious oaths of revenge; and his few pupils and patients were subjected to depressing outpourings about his own ailments. To those physical defects were now added more and more mental disturbances. Voices haunted him, awake and asleep; he complained of a ringing in the ears; he was obsessed by the certainty of approaching death, for his horoscope was unequivocal on that subject. To those who knew him, the eccentricities of a scholar had become the boring rantings of a madman. He was shunned even in the taverns and could no longer rely on an income from gambling. To her great credit, Chiara stood by her son and daughter-in-law and supported them as the money drained away. But Cardano determined that they must move away from Milan, which he saw now only as enemy territory. He finished his book on fate and added the epigraph, "A prophet is not without honour, save in his country, and in his own house".

The choice of venue for his new tussle with misfortune was easily determined. A day's ride from Milan there was a small country town, Gallarate, where lived a cousin, Giocomo Cardano, from whom Gerolamo, at the edge of penury, had borrowed a little money. Giocomo reminded him that at Gallarate there was a castle that was the ancient home of the noble Castillione family, from whom Fazio had been collaterally descended. It seemed sensible to assume, as Giocomo pointed out, that the young doctor and his wife might be better received in Gallarate for his lineage if for nothing else. Surely nothing could be lost, and everything might be gained? After carefully weighing that consideration of family association, frail though it might be, Cardano records, "I resolved to go to Gallarate so that I might have the enjoyment of four other advantages that it offered. First, that in the more healthy air of the country I might shake off entirely the many afflictions to which my flesh succumbed and which were worsened by the foetid air of the plague-ridden city. Secondly that I might earn something by my profession because I would be able to practice. Thirdly, that there would be no need for my spirit to waste while I watched those physicians, by whom I reckoned I had been despoiled, flourishing in wealth and in the high estimation of all men. Lastly, that by following a more frugal way of life, I might make what I possessed last the longer. For all things are cheaper in the country because they do not have to be carried thither, as they do to the towns, and many necessaries may be had for the asking. Persuaded by these arguments, I went to this place."[5]

It was then April 1533 and Lucia was again pregnant, and again she miscarried—probably with the effort of the journey, which was arduous and had to be made on foot because the only two mules they had been able to borrow carried the few possessions they had salved from the sale-room or the pawn-broker. It could scarcely be called a hopeful beginning, but for once Cardano seems not to have buried his natural stoicism beneath mountains of self-pity. Chiara, visiting them in the affluence of rents from her house, which she had apparently let as a brothel,[6] found her daughter-in-law recovering and her son glowing with affection—not only for Lucia but also for a new-found friend, Filippo Archinto, who had allowed Cardano the use of a suite of rooms in his summer house at Gallarate. "My son is pleased because he has found one who has offered him work," she wrote to her agent in Milan; "and also because his own health is much improved."[7] She herself was pleased because, although she had journeyed from Milan with the entire purpose of grandiloquently rescuing Gerolamo and Lucia from the squalor of poverty, she had no need, in the event, to dip into her swelling purse. On the contrary, she could enjoy a few days with them as a guest, noting with the inquisitiveness common in mothers-in-law the methods of household management used by the convalescent Lucia, and preparing herself to act as the envoy of her son's forthcoming fame—of which, she wrote, "I am certain".

Though she was, in that prophecy, to be proved right, her maternal enthusiasm was somewhat ahead of the justifying facts. Cardano was to find Gallarate as unproductive of medical success as had been Sacco and Milan—though for the better reason that the clear air and insular topography of the little town encouraged good health and there were few who needed the services of a doctor. His work for Archinto was of the merest hack nature. The young nobleman was an enthusiastic amateur astronomer and wished to present his opinions in that science to the scholarly world in which it was embraced. But he had no gift for turning his thoughts into words and had offered Cardano a handsome fee to be the "ghost" who directed his pen. It was a task that Cardano found congenial and simple, though he approached it in great earnest and suggested many improvements which Archinto accepted not only with grace but with declared admiration for his mentor's grasp of the whole science. "Here is a genius," Archinto wrote, "who in the extent of his learning has outwritten Galen and dwelt upon the secrets of the skies; knows of numbers as much as any man; delights in music and performs it with grace; can spend upon philosophy great argument; and in the little time when he might be idle puts down notations and sketches of many ingenious engines and toys."[8] The eulogy was in substance true. Cardano had not "outwritten" Galen, the Greek doctor who in the 2nd century wrote more than five hundred works which dominated medicine for centuries: but he had learnt from that prince of physicians anatomy, physiology, pathology, and teleology, and had used Galen's works as a basis for his own youthfully exuberant stricture *On The Differing Opinions of Physicians*. As for mathematics, he was certainly skilled beyond any ordinary person's provenance; and in philosophy he could, and did, argue with logic and force, as he did in most things. Music we know was his great pleasure, and if his own assumptions of competence have up to now seemed a little boastful, it is a happy thing to have them confirmed by his patron. The most interesting observation Archinto makes is upon Cardano's continual jotting down of sketches and ideas for "ingenious engines and toys". The period of his mechanical inventions and his many books of what today would be called "popular science", still lay some years ahead. But it is evident from what Archinto notes that ideas and embryos were even then occupying his capacious mind.

It was ironical that at the very time when Cardano's stars

seemed to favour him, and the Eumenides to have forsaken
their vengeful schemes to punish whatever crimes may have
been committed by the ancestors of his dynasty, the course of
his fortune should have been forced, as it might have been by
some gibing quasi-Procrustes, to remain at its nadir. But so it
was. Archinto was suddenly conscripted into one of the many
campaigns of the Holy League against the Emperor Charles V
and left Gallarate literally in the middle of the night and in the
middle of a long discussion with Cardano on eclectics. The
messenger brought with him the peremptory sealed command of
the Holy League's forces' leader and the young nobleman was
forced to obey. He promised to make provision for Cardano
while he was away; but either his instructions to his lawyer
miscarried or the lawyer enriched himself at Cardano's expense.
However it was, Cardano was deprived of his patron's support
and had to leave the comfortable lodging provided for him. He
once again had to fall back on the gaming table for his earnings; but they amounted to very little. His fortunes were at their
nadir indeed, for it was winter, there was little to be had for the
mere labour of gathering it from the fields, and Lucia was once
more pregnant. "My only advantage was that I was good in
health and my wife with me, and we were able to endure the
winter on the simplest of food and take heart from the fires of
the few friends who would entertain us. At this time I was never
desolate in spirit, though I had lost at the games even my wife's
small jewels and our very bed and accounted that, apart from
the fees of Filippo Archinto, I had earned less than forty crowns
during the whole of my stay at Gallarate."

His cousin Giocomo had clearly been wrong in assuming that
he would gain any mercenary advantage from his Castillione
descent. The castle that had once been the ancestral home had
passed into the hands of another family in payment of a gambling debt; and though the name Castillione still rang with regal
authority through the countryside, the rustic population were
unimpressed by Cardano's remote connexion with that name—
particularly as his station was clearly no more than that of a
hired scribe in the service of Archinto. The breadth of his learning meant nothing to them, for their lives were filled with the
husbandry of their crops and their minds with the earthy wis-

dom of country people. The sophistication of science was to
them quite foreign.

Cardano's good spirits at this luckless time were maintained
by his belief that he would shortly be famous. "Though I may
have but a few years to live, I hear continual voices and dream
visions promising fame. I am content in those. I believe too that
the trinity of Lucia's pregnancies will be fruitful, for there is a
sacred quality in this number." Thus he wrote to his mother at
the beginning of May 1534. Ten days later Lucia successfully
gave birth to a son. The boy was small, weak, and deformed by
a slight curvature of the spine and by having two toes on the
left foot joined together. The midwife was as gloomy about its
survival as had been her counterpart at Gerolamo's own birth.
But Gerolamo, who tenderly attended Lucia at the birth and
staunched a post-natal haemorrhage by the skilful use of some
coagulant which he forgets to describe, was more optimistic.
"But had I known then," he writes forty years later, "of the
wickedness that was to seize the boy and the evil that he was to
cast upon other people, I might in my anguish have been tempted to cast him aside and let him pule in vain. Only at his
baptism did I receive sign that I should be humbled in my joy
in my firstborn. On that day when he was named Giovanni
Battista, the sun shone brightly into the bed-chamber; it was
between the hours of eleven and twelve in the forenoon; and
according to custom we were gathered round the mother's bed.
The curtain was drawn away from the window to let in light
and air. Suddenly a great wasp flew into the room, though it
was by no means the season for wasps, and circled angrily
round the child. We beat it away in fear that it would harm
him with its poison, and it flew angrily against the wall and for
some moments continued a resounding noise like a drum. The
creature disappeared as suddenly as it had come, no one seeing
its departure although all eyes were upon it; and I was filled
with horror by the menacing premonition that a spell was cast
upon my son by an evil insect, and that though its sting had not
afflicted him it had through the powers of darkness poisoned his
spirit."

Of the innumerable premonitions that Cardano experienced
throughout his life, that one was to be mercilessly fulfilled.

7

1535-1536

Soon after the birth of Giovanni, Cardano fell ill with tertian fever. The spasmodic high temperatures lasted for a month, each third day with its "agues and vomitings" leaving him so weak and distressed that he could not rise for ten minutes from his bed "without collapsing like a new born kitten on the floor". He treated himself with cold compresses on the head and at the armpits and drank as much as he dared of some astringent drug which he calls "the Saracen draught", the nature of which remains mysterious. (There was a "Saracen ointment" introduced into Europe at the time of the Crusades, compounded of mercury and animal fat and used in the treatment of syphilis; but mercury taken internally could hardly have helped.) Whatever the draught was—and it was most probably distilled from wormwood or some other herb with tonic properties—its purpose, says Cardano, was "to dry up the abhorrent liquors deriving from the poison".[1]

During the month of his illness he was reduced to complete destitution because of his inability to earn even the paltry sums he might have got by gaming or by treating the few sick people to be found in Gallarate. Chiara had for the time being turned against him after a quarrel over the naming of the child, and Cardano was in any case too obstinate to look to her for help. So, "like a man hemmed in upon a barren rock who resolves to cast himself into the sea, I resolved to quit Gallarate and return to Milan, which in my bones I had always thought to be the first scene of my fame".

Carrying the wallet containing his few medical instruments and his supply of powders and potions, and with his books piled on a flat wheeled trolley pulled behind them, he and Lucia set

out once again for Milan at the end of August 1534. They had
no money to hire horses, or even for food, and they had to beg
for alms and sleep in the fields for three days and nights. Cardano seems to have had no plans to put into operation when
they reached the city: had he not said, indeed, that he was only
casting himself from a barren rock into a merciless sea? But
since he also said that he had been lured back by his faith
in his own eventual fame, he presumably felt that his fortunes
were about to change. His premonitions, like life itself, were
ever contradictory. For the moment, however, there were no
signs of fame even seeking him out, let alone settling herself
upon him. The unprepossessing appearance of the ragged
couple and their sickly child attracted only charges of vagrancy.
As they begged for alms in the streets of one of the richest cities
in Europe they were driven aside and spat upon with a vehe-
ment contempt almost equal to that bestowed on lepers. Filthy
and starving, they found their way after some weeks of wretchedness and anguish to the public poorhouse, still grandly
known as the xenodochium from the Greek institutions dedicated to Jovi Xenio, but now little more than a squalid patrimony of the Church. They sheltered from October until the end
of the year. Both he and Lucia were committed to the most
menial tasks to qualify for their subsistence. It was as if charity
could be dispensed only in marriage with humiliation, quite
bereft of compassion. But to this period of extreme poverty
Cardano brought a dignity that proved the dichotomy of his
character. In real crises his self-pity was subdued by determination, he drew from misfortune a strength remarkable among so
many weaknesses, real and imagined. "I am hot-tempered, rude,
vindictive," he wrote of himself; "I am prone to vice and ill-
doing. But I am also timid, I forego opportunities for revenge
that are offered me. I let my face contradict my thoughts. I am
sometimes silent, sometimes talkative. My gait is irregular: I
move sometimes quickly, sometimes slowly. I am affectionate,
but I am also reckless in speech and injure those whom I love
unwittingly. I am a worshipper of fame and thrust aside the
commonplace; but still, knowing how great may be the power
of little things at any moment in the course of an undertaking, I
remember everything that may be useful."[2]

At the end of the year Cardano had a typically mysterious encounter with a wizard, a wild creature who, like Cardano, had been admitted to the poorhouse in a state of destitution. The skill in necromancy which he claimed, he claimed privily, for a wizard is only the male counterpart of a witch and the horrors of the *Malleus Maleficarum* would have been invoked if the ecclesiastics of the establishment had had the mildest suspicion that they were harbouring such a creature. But he attached himself to Cardano and urged him to accept the advantage of having the ill-spells released from him. Ever curious in all things and by no means afraid of extending his knowledge of the occult, Cardano willingly accepted the offer. It was a traumatic experience, as he tells us years later. "I was given first a great purge of the herb Demonifuge; then my flesh was pounded beneath stones which left no bruises but which, my benefactor said, were grinding the bones of the devil that lurked within me and if I would but listen I would hear the screams from the tortured thing. There was, in truth, a great ringing in my ears such as I had suffered for many years; but it is also true that from that time forth I never experienced that ringing again. So who is to say it was not the sound of the demon within me being driven from me? Nor was that all. Nearby the hospice was a pool that had all the signs of remaining stagnant for many years. Toads leapt upon its edge and the plants and weeds on its surface were of a glutinous kind with slime. Here I had to go at night with my benefactor, a full moon being reflected precisely in the centre of the pool, and immerse my head where the moon lay, while all the vapours of the spell of which I was victim were drawn upward to the atmosphere of that nearest and most benign of the planets, accompanied by an incantation of extraordinary words of which I could hear only the harmony, so to speak, and no particular notes. After this I was to dry my head on unfouled straw from a nearby byre and reward my benefactor with a pouch of powdered alicorn,* which I did and

---

* The horn of that fabulous creature the unicorn, supposed to be an antidote to any poison, just as rhinocerous horn is supposed to be an aphrodisiac. These curious tusks, with their familiar spiral striations, exist in profusion and are often venerated by churches for their symbolic holiness. Most evidence suggests that they are in fact the tusks of narwhals. But no one has yet explained how the relicts of exclusively arctic creatures

completed my release from bondage to ill fortune. From that time forward, this strange necromancer told me, I should fare famously. And I have no cause to declare him false."[3]

Cardano speaks there with some reserve. Clearly the scientific side of his mind is at variance with the inborn superstitions of the age. But whether or not the wizard can be credited with the change, Cardano's life was shortly afterward diverted along a different course. Early in 1535 Filippo Archinto returned from active service and at once established his protégé in one of his own houses; but with respect for Cardano's independence of spirit he also arranged for him to earn the money to pay the rent and support Lucia and the child. However, even Archinto's influence was not powerful enough to overcome the College of Physicians' resistance to Cardano's membership. But there was a most suitable vacancy in a public lectureship under the endowment of one of the past governors of the xenodochium, and Archinto nominated Cardano for the post. The lecturer was called upon to discourse on geometry, arithmetic, and astronomy, plus other subjects to be chosen by himself. The lectures were to be given only on public holidays, so no great demands were made on time; and although the stipened was small—seven crowns a year—the prestige attaching to the post was considerable and attracted many fee-paying pupils.[4] Cardano wisely realized the need to make the lectures appealing; and within a few months he had established himself as a forceful and entertaining lecturer with the gift of clarity. To the three set studies he had added architecture and geography and these popular subjects gained him further pupils. Preparing his lectures gave him the idea of writing books on all five subjects, and he set about them at once. True, he had as yet no publisher, and seems not to have sought one. But the long spell of relative idleness and despondency had left him with an insatiable urge to work. His income during 1535 amounted to fifty crowns: no great fortune, but enough to establish a household of a nurse for Giovanni, two servants, and a mule. During the year Chiara, with whom he had now made up his quarrel, came to live with

---

found their way to medieval Europe from regions unknown, let alone explored.

him and Lucia, bringing with her her sister Margarita. She must also have brought some contribution to the household expenses, for twenty of the fifty crowns went in servants' wages and the remainder would certainly not have covered the rent, taxes, and food for eight people. Even with Chiara's help the household was much grander than Cardano should have maintained at that time. But the women pressed him into living above his income, and, like his father, he could not be bothered to take any interest in money matters. The line of least resistance was to let them have their own way. Argumentative and truculent though he could be, he needed peace for his work; and if it could be gained by so simple a course as withdrawing from household affairs, then there lay his choice. His own needs were modest. His breakfast was invariably gruel made of barley bread and water or goat's milk flavoured with nasturtium leaves, rue, or parsley; for his dinner he might have a baked fish or a plate of stewed meat. Wine was the only palatable drink and he drank it copiously; but then so did everybody else, perhaps subconsciously understanding the dangers of water polluted by sewage and rats. He had only two extravagances : books and writing materials; and in both he took immense pleasure. Though it could hardly be called an extravagance, he also found great pleasure in the company of animals. Cats, dogs, storks and mules were about the house whenever the family was suitably lodged. "They demand nothing," he wrote, "and their presence steadies the spirit." One of them, it is worth noting in passing, also caused him considerable trouble. He had just completed his small book on geography, which was based on Ptolemy's work with the light of later knowledge shed upon it, when his cat Orlando came upon the manuscript on the work table and, pleased by the crackling noise made by the paper, tore almost every sheet to shreds. The whole thing had to be rewritten. "But I learned from this," Cardano says philosophically, "that a cat is a creature of of the suddenest tempers; for I had left Orlando curled tightly in sleep when I left the chamber for no more than to seek a book in another room; he must have sprung instantly to action as I left, perhaps in his feline way disapproving of either my style or my project."[5]

Many others more influential than Orlando the cat were to disapprove of Cardano, his style, his projects, his temper, his morals. Certainly from 1535 the course of his fortune changed for the better. But fortune is always relative. There were many hazards to be met.

8

1536–1537

The student Ottaviano Scoto, whom Cardano had befriended at Pavia and whom he had not seen for ten years, suddenly looms importantly in his life. Scoto is on a visit to Milan from his home in Venice and attends one of Cardano's lectures. The two renew old acquaintance, Scoto reminding Cardano of his letter declaring his longing to return to Pavia and enjoy the tranquillity of the university and the friendship of his fellow student. (The plague and the battle of Pavia had intervened and the friendship had been interrupted.) "And now, my good friend," says Scoto, "you have become a great and famous man offering dissertations on sphere and circles and interpreting Euclid for such as me who have no brain to speak of, having done nothing more startling than inherit the printing-office of his father."[1]

Disabusing Scoto of the notion that he is famous, Cardano is none the less immediately on the alert. Surprisingly for him, usually so slow to grasp matters of commerce, he sees to the heart of the main chance. A printer! Can he persuade Scoto to undertake publication of one or more of the manuscripts on which he has spent so much time? He hesitates for fear that such a rapid approach will seem too full of vulgar self-interest. "To leap upon my friend's good nature would have seemed no more than the wheedling of a money-grubber".[2] On the other hand, he could not bear to let pass an opportunity which, he is certain, has been revealed to him in a recent dream. "In that vision," he says, "I beheld my self running toward the base of a mountain which stood upon my right hand, in company with a vast crowd of people of every age and station, poor and rich, clad in every kind of raiment. I enquired whither we were all going and one of the multitude cried that we were all hastening toward death. I was greatly alarmed at these words and turned about, only to find before me another slope covered with vines bare of both leaves and grapes, as we commonly see them in autumn. I grasped the vines and began to ascend. At first I found this difficult, for the slope was very steep; but having surmounted it I made my way more easily, though I was forced to take great care, for steep naked rocks were on every side and many times I narrowly escaped falling from a great height into a gloomy chasm. At last there appeared before me a wide plain barren of all save stunted trees and steamy swamps. Making my way across this in continual alarm I came at last to a small hut thatched with reeds and straw. And there I met a boy, no more than twelve years old, clad in a grey cloak, whose hand I grasped as I woke from sleep sweating with terror."[3]

It is fully in character that Cardano should see in this dream the allegory of his life. The upward climb, the barren rocks and chasms, the vines autumnally bare but secretly holding the sap and promise of spring, the hut offering rest after an arduous journey, the child who would carry the name of Cardano onward like a torch illuminating with fame the dark passages of the future. Scoto's fortuitous reappearance fully fledged as a printer could scarcely be anything but an opportunity to be grasped. "If my chart told truthfully and I had but a decade of my life to span, then I must neglect the courtesies of friendship and press my suit for Ottaviano's favour."[4]

In the event he had no need to swallow his pride and speak on his own behalf. As if under command of the fortunate spirit within whose ambiance Cardano for the time being stood, Scoto asked him outright for the honour of printing the next Cardano book. He was astonished to learn that so far not a word of any of his friend's numerous manuscripts had appeared in print. "Joyfully he said that he would take all the risk of publication, and that even if he were to lose by it, it would be small cost for the privilege of being the first to put Doctor Cardano into the vision of the public."[5]

The choice of manuscript now had to be made. There were pamphlets, treatises, whole books and unfinished books. He was himself surprised to find he had written so much—"Always in the hope of publication but never with the slightest effort on my

part to induce any printer to take upon himself such a sorry
burden." He could now show the world his explorations of
geometry, arithmetic, architecture, geography, gambling, medicine. But which? Begging Scoto to let him consider the proposi-
tion seriously, he engaged to hand over the manuscript of his
choice a week hence. He then retired to his workroom and
"after many hours of doubt" decided to present to the world
through Scoto's good offices a rewritten version of the treatise he
had written while still a student *On The Differing Opinions of
Physicians*. Since that work, taken into consideration with his
bastardy and aggressive manner, had been the root cause of his
exclusion from the College of Physicians, its choice may seem a
stupid flaunting of bitterness in the face of transiently smiling
fortune. But as with his inference of literal truth from the allegory of the dream, the choice was completely in character. First,
he recognized that medicine was his chief love and that all the
public attention he had so far gained had been directed at his
other studies. "Whatever small fame I had achieved in Milan as
geometer, astronomer, designer, interpreter of Euclid, astrologer,
geographer—this was of less import to me than my true voca-
tion, where my reputation had scarcely begun."[6] Secondly, he
had in mind the dealing of a swingeing blow at the establishment of the College and could see that it could best be dealt by
the caustic comments he was prepared to add to his student
thesis. In a single week he rewrote and added what was necessary and handed the new manuscript to Scoto. It was called
now *On the Bad Practice of Medicine in Common Use* and
Scoto returned to Venice promising to put it through the press
with all speed. He would personally see to the proof reading and
thereby save time in transmission to and from Milan. Neither he
nor Cardano realized what seeds of disaster lay in that kindly
intended offer.

The book was published early in 1536 and was an immediate
success so far as concerned the ordinary public. For a doctor to
pick fault with his colleagues gave the lay reader a sense of
identification, a feeling that here was a spokesman for him,
putting into words that had the backing of esoteric knowledge
the very doubts that the plain man invariably felt when faced
with the opinions of medical men who surrounded themselves

with impenetrable mysteries and could cure no one without consulting with others of their kin who also demanded fees for their contributions to grave arguments at the bedside. The common medical practices that Cardano vehemently denounced were seventy-two in number. He attacked first of all the principle that in every case of illness immediate recourse should be had to powders and potions. "To do nothing with physic is far better than to do too much, and a physician desiring to act rightly should consider a great number of things before setting down prescriptions for the pharmacist to manufacture." The prevailing belief that there lurked among the pharmacist's phials and mortars a single remedy for all sicknesses was also blisteringly attacked. He declared utter nonsense the practice of denying wine and fish to those with fevers, and accused of murderous intent those who refused to bleed a patient suffering acute pain from inflammation of the peritoneum. These and the other three score and more of medical errors he denounced were, he wrote, "the result of the tribal insecurities of men who banded themselves together and showed to the world a surface of pomp and learning that satisfactorily concealed from the beholders the depth of ignorance beneath".

It was scarcely surprising that such a book should immediately arouse the violent antagonism of the College of Physicians. That was Cardano's intention. But he had himself put into his enemies' hands the very weapons to repulse his attack. Haste on his part to get the book rewritten, and the absence of opportunity to correct the proofs, had resulted in barbarous errors of grammar and syntax as well as errors of fact; and Scoto's compositors had composed innumerable misprints in the text, which Scoto, if he had read the proofs at all, had failed to correct. Looking back on the book from his mature years, Cardano groaned, as has many an author since, at his own rashness. "I blush to acknowledge that there were more than even three hundred blunders of mine in this book, exclusive of misprints. And I long since had it in my mind to blot it out from the number of my offspring : but to that course there was the objection of a certain special usefulness connected with it, by which it had been made so saleable that in its second year the printer would have issued it again to the public if I had not resisted his desire."[7] The immediate result of publication was devastating. Of the attacks he had made against the established medical profession, the doctors sarcastically said that a man who wrote about *The Bad Practice of Medicine in Common Use* should have a practice of his own to prove his experience. Nor did they fail to advertise the fact that he had been excluded from membership of the College of Physicians. Could the public not clearly see that his very eccentricities would preclude his membership, and that his so-called treatments would imperil the lives of any patients foolish enough to put themselves in his hands? He was a young man who lectured on astronomy, geography, arithmetic, and architecture; he knew nothing of the practice of medicine and his academic qualifications were dubious to say the least—for had not the voting on his graduation twice been against him? The truth was, that he was filled with envy at the success of doctors who had absorbed the collective learning of the ages and thought to strike at them with the puny blows of inexperience. And he had not even mastered the art of expressing himself, for many of his sentences were incomprehensible. "All this," Cardano wrote sadly, "resulted from a book written and printed with so much hope of happy issue. It was to have led the way to sick-beds, by the proof it would afford that he who wrote it had thought soundly and deeply as a practical physician. It was to have brought me the first honours of public authorship; but where I sowed for honour I reaped nothing but shame. The book damaged me in every respect save one: it sold in great quantities because it was bought to be abused. My friend Scoto rejoiced; but I grieved."[8]

He need not have grieved quite so blackly. The number bought to be abused by the defenders of the citadel of the establishment was far exceeded by the number bought by the lay public—who, as I have said, were delighted to be able to identify themselves with a spokesman who clearly found great fault among the mysteries of medicine.

So, although Cardano's attack on the citadel was repulsed, he had found, but for the present unknowingly, on another flank, reinforcements who would serve him well.

9

1537–1541

He saw himself defeated, believed himself vanquished, and sank
again into the depths of self-pity. He must have been a great
trial to his family; and Lucia, who was again pregnant and
herself suffering from bouts of depression, wrote feelingly to
Archinto asking him to come and comfort her husband "who at
this time is of a melancholy that makes me fear for him".[1]
Archinto came at once. His concern for his friend was touching.
Although a year younger than Cardano, he adopted the attitude
of an old, wise, and sympathetic counsellor. "He alone of those
who knew me," says Cardano, "could rouse me from my
lethargy with hope."[2] But it was something more practical than
hope that Archinto this time brought to the despondent doctor.
He had news that one of the patients Cardano had surreptitiously treated before he had moved to Gallarate had fully
recovered and now offered an official appointment. The patient
was Francesco Gaddi, prior of the order of Augustinian Friars
in Milan. He had suffered from a scrofulous infection which
was most probably tuberculoid leprosy. That ancient dread
disease brought little but suspicion and hostility to the unfortunate sufferers, and treatment, or even attempts at treatment, were
almost unknown. Compassion was limited to the occasional
provision of "lazarettes"—refuges for those cast out—and only
quacks would claim to cure the afflicted—sometimes by the
drastic method of branding the patches on the skin with hot
irons. Cardano's treatment of the prior had been simple and
completely untrammelled by medicaments. Upon consideration
of his patient's mode of life, which involved the almost complete
neglect of all bodily needs in the cause of spiritual dedication,
he arrived at the common-sense conclusion that no cure could

be effected on a dirty, under-nourished, body. He sternly told the prior that if he believed his work to be of value to God he should see to it that his body was enabled to continue its function by harbouring his spirit. He prescribed regular hours of sleep and exercise, frequent bathing, the wearing of linen instead of sackcloth next to the skin, and a reasonable diet including fish and wine. Astonishingly, the prior had taken Cardano's advice and had so recovered the health of his body that it had resisted the further attacks of the disease—which, indeed, had withdrawn and left his skin clear and whole. Now he wished to appoint Cardano as official physician to the Priory in acknowledgement of his skill.

"Nothing could have given Cardano greater pleasure," Archinto wrote in his memoirs years later, after he had become successively a Count Palatine, a priest, Governor of Rome, Bishop of Borgo San Sepolcro, and Archbishop of Milan. "Gaddi was his first notable patient. The appointment was worth scarcely anything in money, but it carried prestige and set my friend in a position where he could thumb his nose at the Milan College, for not even the most skilled of their number had been able to bring relief to Gaddi."[3]

Although Cardano was now well placed for a new and potentially more effective attack upon the College, he withheld his fire—either from indifference or because he shrewdly realized that delay until he had built up a practice would bring him even stronger armaments. He had certainly not forgotten that when playing chess, cards, and dice in the taverns he had publicly sworn oaths of revenge upon the College. But his malice was not impatient. Nor was it specially violent. In any case, he suddenly had much to occupy his medical attention. His prescription books for the years 1536 to 1539, and his memoirs and other autobiographical works show that his appointment to the priory was of great value as a commendation for his medical reliability. The chagrin of the College doctors was great, but they could not prevent him from practicing, for he had his degree. And now there was no need for him to seek his patients surreptitiously : they came to him.

His successes were often remarkable. There was a woman called Martha Mott who for thirteen years had suffered from an ulcerated leg and general wasting of the body and had been bedridden in consequence. Within two years Cardano had restored her to a healthy state with nothing but a slight limp to remind her of her previous sorry condition. He was equally successful with Tibbold, a baker who suffered from what was apparently tuberculosis and whom he advised to give up the floury, overheated bakehouse and substitute for it the strong country air of Gallarate with plenty of rest, a light nourishing diet, and interests undemanding of energy. It was sensible treatment, and Tibbold recovered to the extent of ceasing to cough up blood and sputum. Encouraged by this success, Cardano sought out other consumptives and prescribed the same treatment—always "within the clear air of Gallarate". In doing so he was establishing the principle of the sanatorium—which was to be rediscovered three hundred years later and to remain standard treatment for tuberculosis until our own day. His rivals were furious and fell upon him with accusations of quackery, since they could not believe that the simplicity of his treatment of a disease which for countless centuries had been embedded in superstition could be effective. Watching like vultures, they spotted a couple of cases of failure and immediately bruited these abroad and waited to settle on the dying reputation of the man they feared. But Cardano's reputation was not so easily assailed. He pointed out with acerbity that one of the failures was a man who had gone straight from church to a gaming tavern through a rainstorm and had remained all night in wet clothes; the other was one who, having been caught in the act of burglary, had jumped through a window into a fish pond. In both cases, understandably, death followed a recurrence of the malady. The College vultures retired from their watchful perches unsatisfied. And gradually they were forced to relinquish their hopes of pickings from the corpse of Cardano's reputation. On the contrary, they were shortly to be forced to pick, instead, at humble pie. Donato Lanza, a pharmacist who often made up Cardano's prescriptions, had been cured by him of an affliction of the eyes and in consequence held his benefactor to be the most eminent of doctors. So it was not surprising that he should be loud in his praises at every opportunity. One such opportunity occurred when a rich senator of Cremona, Francisco Sfondrato, was discussing the mysterious illness of his young son, a child of ten months, who had suddenly been afflicted with convulsions and rigidity of the neck. Sfondrato agreed to call Cardano for a consultation with his own doctors, both of whom were consultants at the College—one of them being also the procurator. The other was the senior imperial physician. Their names were Luca della Croce and Ambrose Cavenega. No doubt they would have refused to consult with Cardano had Sfondrato not been such an eminent man and one who could easily have brought them to book for neglect of duty; but in the circumstances they came sheepishly to the child's bedside. Ethics demanded that Cardano should examine and diagnose first, leaving the final pronouncement to the senior doctor. "They stood by," says Cardano, "their sneers scarcely concealed by their beards, and waited to rip my conclusions to pieces." They were disappointed. Cardano gently examined the baby, found that its neck seemed to be forcibly held back by some unnatural tension of the muscles, and after a while said: "This is a clear case of opisthotonos".* Cavenega simply looked blank, betraying his ignorance; but Della Croce had the grace to praise Cardano's discernment and asked if he knew the remedy. Whereupon Cardano reeled off many aphorisms of Hippocrates concerning the treatment of convulsions. Both doctors realized that if they were to argue and be proved wrong they would lose face; they therefore played their only card, which was to leave the case to Cardano. He ordered that the child's wet nurse should eat no meat while she was feeding him, which he claimed would improve the quality of her milk, and that fomentations of linseed oil and oil of lilies should be applied hourly to the child's neck and shoulders. "The senator drew me aside," Cardano wrote, "and told me, 'I give you this child as a son. Consider him your own and do with him as you would your own child. Do not concern yourself about the other doctors. Let them be offended if they will'. I told him that the issue of the treatment could only be doubtful. But they followed it, and within four days the child had improved and in due course

---

* Muscular spasms causing the neck or limbs to be forced backward; a form of tetanus.

recovered. From that time on Sfondrato was a faithful patron and a good patient."[4]

Having thus been forced to acknowledge Cardano's talents, the faculty of the College had no course but to think again about his admission. They made their deliberations long and grave, mainly to convince themselves that they had something to deliberate about. "In the end," Cardano says wryly, "they were compelled to sully their respectability by welcoming into their company an ill-born scholar. So it came about that in the year 1539, after twelve years of resolute exclusion, I was enrolled among the Milanese College of Physicians and was granted the lawful right to practice for fees or to take office as a teacher of Medicine in that city."[5]

Much had happened in Cardano's life between the publication of *The Bad Practice of Medicine* and his election to membership of the College besides the acquisition of patients and the spreading of his reputation. He was never a man to be idle; and a few patients, gradually come by, left him plenty of time for thought and work. To improve his Latin style he read the entire works of Cicero. (His prose never achieved gracefulness or indeed any other distinction; but it became workmanlike and clear.) He studied Greek, French, and Spanish with the object of being able to read in those languages rather than to converse in them. And of course he wrote. For although his first publication had brought him, as he thought, little but derision, he was constitutionally a scholar and perforce needed to set down his thoughts and studies, even without the hope of publication.

Two short works belonging to this time were written at the instance of Archinto, who had fallen into great favour with the pope, Paul III, and was about to take holy orders and receive his appointment as Apostolic Protonotary and Governor of Rome. Archinto sent Cardano an urgent letter saying that the pope was "vastly interested" in astronomy and astrology and that short treatises on these subjects could well please the Holy Father and bring Cardano to his notice. Cardano at once set to and produced a paper somewhat challengingly entitled *Emendation of the Celestial Movements*, and another which was nothing less than a life of Jesus Christ based on His horoscope.

In view of Archinto's counsel the subjects were sensibly chosen; and Archinto's sponsorship was reinforced by that of the French ambassador at the papal court, Marshal Brissac; so Cardano had every reason to believe that a journey to Rome to present his works to His Holiness would be well worth while. He made the journey, but characteristically was in no mind to fawn upon the Holy Father for his favour. Rather the opposite, in fact; for he hated unctuousness and rather than risk any evidence of it he attended the papal court bristling with argument. In the event, he might have saved himself the trouble. His books were accepted by a minor official who evidently thought better of advancing the ungainly and aggressive doctor's steps into the presence of His Holiness, and he was given his congé. He was not disappointed. He had planned only to present the books to the pope with scholarly respect and perhaps to argue on the subject matter. Any favour that would make the journey worth while could only come from the pope's reading of them and possible approval of the scholarship revealed in them. Well, the pope had the books: no doubt in due course he would read and remark upon them. Cardano returned to Milan unaffected by his cursory dismissal. No dream or other portent gave him any warning of the punitive reward that years later was to fall upon him for his horoscope of Christ.

Nor had he any intimation of the wretched outcome of another event that gave him great happiness at the time: the birth of his daughter. She was born soon after the publication of *The Bad Practice of Medicine* when he was in the state of depression that caused Lucia to send for Archinto. She was a fine healthy child and he writes of her birth that "It was accomplished with the greatest of ease", and of the child herself that, "She was in no way disfigured as was our firstborn, nor was her baptism marked by any untoward incident". She was baptised in the name of Chiara to please Cardano's mother, who was at that time in a decline of health that made her bedridden and to whom he wrote tenderly, "It is a signal of our affection for you that our daughter should be as you in name and our plea to the spirits of fortune that she maybe likewise of your character." Perhaps Cardano should have been more specific in his plea; for the child inherited only the licentiousness of her grandmother's nature. But at the time she naturally enough revealed nothing of her inheritance and gave her parents only intense pleasure.

Less than a year later, Cardano, in numinous mood, hears a mysterious tapping, "As of drops of water upon the pavement", followed by "A heavy sound as of the unloading of a wagonful of planks which caused the bed to tremble"; both of which noises he interprets as portents of his mother's approaching death. And indeed she died a few hours later. But tappings and tremblings of the bed regardless, her death could hardly have been unexpected, since she was old and had been in failing health for some time. Cardano immediately inherited the house she died in, for, unlike her husband Fazio, whose patrimony was still the subject of seemingly endless legal wrangles, she was businesslike enough to make her intentions regarding the disposal of her hereditaments incontrovertibly clear in a will properly signed and witnessed. She also left to her son some money, the sum of which he avoids mentioning—either because he thought the matter unimportant, or because he was surprised at the meanness of her gift and wished to spare her the sneers of those who might observe it. The former seems more probable, his indifference to money being so notable.

Possibly because of the rather grand house Chiara had left him (it had been bought with the income from her brothels), and his appointment as physician to the Augustinians, he was offered the Chair of Medicine at his *alma mater*, Pavia. But the university had even then not recovered from the economic ruin forced upon it by the war of 1525, and though admittedly uninterested in money, Cardano was not quite so uninterested that he would take an appointment that promised no payment at all. He had, in any case, many projects in mind that, with his growing practice, would leave him too little time for a regular stint of teaching. He rejected the offer.

One of the projects he wanted to begin was a book on arithmetic—not a book for the expert like himself but for the ordinary man for whom figures and algebraic equations were a mysterious forest through which there was no well lighted path. He planned the work with exemplary thoroughness, describing first what each of its sixty-eight chapters should contain and making of that prospectus a chapter in itself. The actual treatment was equally thorough and considerate of the inexpert reader's need to have explained to him the elementary operations of arithmetic before going on to such calculations as those involving combined integers and fractions; to kalends, nones, ides, and cycles; to the natural and supernatural properties of numbers; to the rules of mensuration; and to higher mathematical discussions. He had reached that part of the book dealing with advanced matters when he entered upon a quarrel with another scholar that was to become famous in the annals of mathematics.

The custom in those days was for scholars to correspond with each other regarding matters in their published works by way of an intermediary bookseller. Booksellers were often journeymen printers (and publishers as well) and their travels formed a convenient linkage between the cities, while their reasonably comprehensive minds, developed by the variety of subjects in the books they sold, could cope adequately with the details of scholarly messages and queries. Cardano had heard of two mathematicians, Tartaglia and Fiore, who had been engaged in dispute over an algebraic problem. Many of the rules of algebra were then unknown; and indeed mathematicians had not yet arrived at the fact that the resolution of all cases of an algebraic problem may be comprehended in a simple formula, which may be obtained from a single case, merely by changing the signs. The intense and widespread interest in mathematical matters was, on a smaller scale, equivalent to that shown in our own day by the scientists concerned with space travel. Then, as now, interest in such matters overcame even political, religious, or other forms of strife, and the advancement of learning was hastened. The two disputants in this case, Tartaglia and Fiore, were both Venetians who had been engaged in a match of algebraic knowledge in which each posed the other a number of questions which could only be answered by the formulation of a new rule. The match was backed by a wager to give it the spice of personal interest—the wager being that the loser should buy the winner an elaborate supper—and it had been won by Tartaglia, who had hit upon the rule for solving a case of complex cubic equation and had, naturally, put to his opponent questions that were unanswerable except by that rule. Accepting defeat with good grace, Fiore had settled his wager and asked to be shown the new rule. But Tartaglia had refused, explaining that he was not prepared to reveal his secret until he had protected it by the 16th-century equivalent of copyright. Such protection could only be secured by applying through countless officials of gradually increasing importance until the request at last reached the emperor himself, who could give or withhold his imprimatur as his interest dictated. The process took time, as Fiore well knew; but he chose to take Tartaglia's refusal as a personal affront, an implication of his intent to plagiarize Tartaglia's discovery, and the two engaged in an intense battle of invective which held public interest for a year or more.

At this stage Cardano entered the scene. He took the view that the protection of personal interests was of less importance than the spread of knowledge. Certainly it was a convenient view to hold at the time, since the development of his own book depended on knowing the very rule that Tartaglia had discovered; but it was in any case characteristic of Cardano that he should put science before self. He communicated with Tartaglia through the customary medium of a bookseller, and the correspondence was recorded in one of Tartaglia's memorandum books. It is headed: "Inquiry made by Zuan Antonio, bookseller, in the name of one Gerolamo Cardano, Physician and Public Reader of Mathematics in Milan", and continues in the form of dialogues.

Antonio. Messer Nicolo Tartaglia, I have been directed to you by a worthy man, a physician of Milan, named Messer Gerolamo Cardano, who is a very great mathematician, and reads Euclid there in Milan publicly, and who is at present causing to be printed a work of his on the Practice of Arithmetic and Geometry and Algebra, which will be of some note. And because he has understood that you have been engaged in disputation with Messer Fiore, putting to him for a wager certain questions that could only be answered by knowing the general rule for resolving the case of the cosa and cube equal to the number, which general rule you had found by your own discovery. Therefore his excellency prays you that you will kindly make known to him that rule discovered by you, and if you think fit will make it public under your name in his present

work, but if you do not think fit that it should be published he
will keep it secret.

Tartaglia. Tell his excellency that he must pardon me; when
I propose to publish my own invention I will publish it in a
work of my own, and not in the work of another man, so that
his excellency must hold me excused.

Antonio. If you object to make known to him your discovery,
his excellency has bidden me pray that you will, however, give
him the said questions that you posed to Fiore, that he may
attempt his own resolution of them.

Tartaglia. Of those (though I can ill spare the time) I will
make a copy. But his excellency, whatever his competence, will
be unable to resolve them, for to do that would mean his excellency had a wit like to my own, which he has not.[7]

This conceited message was received wrathfully by Cardano.
But for the moment he did not reply. Instead, he brooded on
the questions and in a short time had discovered the general
rule that Tartaglia had thought beyond the scope of any mind
but his own. He then sent to Tartaglia a letter. "I wonder
much, dear Tartaglia," he wrote, "at the unhandsome reply you
made to Zuan Antonio, bookseller, who on my part prayed that
you might tell me of your discovery so that the knowledge might
be shared by means of the book I am about to print. It grieves
me much that among other discomforts of this science those who
engage in it are so discourteous, and presume so much on their
own worth, that it is not without reasons that they are called
fools by the surrounding vulgar. I would pluck you out of this
conceit of thinking you are the first great man in the world, and
admonish you that you are nearer to the valley than the mountain top. For what can be done by one can be done by another
of equal or greater merit, and I have myself after some cogita-
tion come upon the method which you thought so secret. Therefore I hold it to be my own discovery, which it is, and I shall
print it in my new work, and gain protection for it from the
Ever August Roman Emperor, Charles the Fifth, though I shall
not omit to publish that you too, Tartaglia, are the discoverer.
So my original purpose is thus achieved, for I wished only to
hasten the dissemination of knowledge, which is for the benefit
of all and not to be nursed as a cipher by a few scholars; and

that purpose might have been served as well, and quicker, had you replied as I asked."[8]

This testy exchange, which seems to be no more than a mild professorial tussle, masked an enmity that was planted then and grew in bitterness. Because of Archinto's influence through the papal court, Cardano obtained copyright protection for his book *The Practice of Arithmetic and Simple Mensuration* long before Tartaglia's application had worked its way up to the emperor. Tartaglia therefore felt justified in accusing Cardano of plagiarism. The branches of the growing enmity were nourished by the poisonous sap of recrimination, and Tartaglia was to prove himself a redoubtable foe. But the crippling blow he dealt Cardano was delayed for some years.

The Practice of Arithmetic, for which Cardano received an advance payment of ten golden crowns, was an immediate success. His publisher this time was a Milan bookseller-cum-printer named Bernardo Caluscho. There had been no quarrel with Scoto, but Cardano had learnt his lesson on the troubles that arise from lack of attention to proof reading, and he personally supervised the production of every page of *The Practice of Arithmetic*—wisely, for it contained many geometrical figures. It also contained an advertisement telling his readers of the many tracts, treatises, and other works he had written and which awaited publication. These numbered thirty-four and included the two manuscripts presently with the pope, the *Life of Christ* in horoscope form and the *Emendation of the Celestial Movements*; there was also a work on judicial astronomy, three volumes of philosophy entitled *Consolatione*, the book on gambling, another philosophical work on wisdom, and a long theological discussion on the *Arcana of Eternity*. It would certainly not be possible to accuse Cardano of idleness during those years before he was elected to the College of Physicians. And now, in 1540, with the publication of *The Practice of Arithmetic*, he was to find the reward of fame, if not yet of money, for his industry.

The triumph of the book was caused by qualities that affect successful book publication in any age: it answered a demand, and it was written in a style suitable for a widespread audience

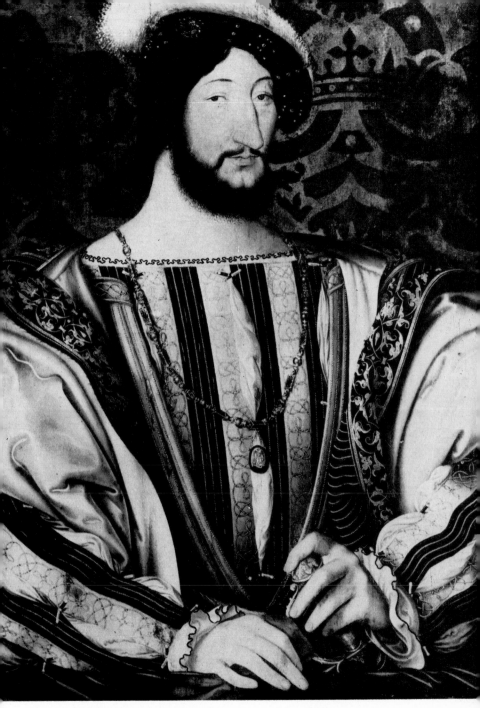

Francis I, who succeeded Louis XII as King of France and became the bitter rival of Charles V in the struggle between France and the Austro-Spanish Habsburgs

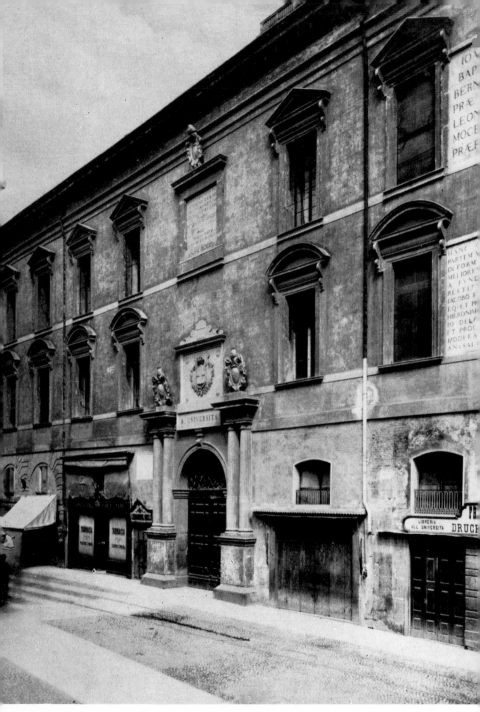

Padua University, where Cardano taught after the Battle of Pavia
in 1525

who had no specialized knowledge. These are hallmarks of popularity.

Slow though communications were, there was no lack of travellers; and the book soon found readers in France, Spain, and Germany. And from Nuremberg there came an offer of a kind so rare as not usually even to enter any author's thoughts. Johannes Petreius, a Nuremberg printer who had read not only the book but the advertisement too, offered to print and publish, on a royalty basis, any unpublished work that Cardano cared to entrust to him. He also offered the services, as editor, of a Nuremberg scholar, Andreas Osiander, who would see everything through the press on Cardano's behalf. It was an irresistible offer and Cardano accepted it at once. "I believed myself to be near death, according to my horoscope, and therefore seized the chance of fame which also was written in the stars." He spent the works on judicial astronomy and gambling for Petreius to be getting on with, and at the same time, remembering his gratitude to his Venice publisher, sent Scoto the philosophical treatise *Consolatione*, which, not being a technical work, was unlikely to suffer importantly from careless proof reading as had *The Bad Practice of Medicine*. Another gesture which marked Cardano's sense of obligation was his dedication of the arithmetic book to Francesco Gaddi, his first notable patient. "I wished," he wrote, "to ensure that the epoch of fame I was now entering, should be shared by those who contributed to it."[9]

But though the fame came quickly, money to match it did not—except to Caluscho, publisher of the book, whose ten crowns given to Cardano as a speculative venture were soon multiplied a hundredfold. But Cardano had no cause for complaint—nor did he make any. He had been glad enough to accept the money and was himself shrewd enough to descry Caluscho's greater shrewdness in recognizing the merit of the work and foreseeing its popular appeal. And in any case Cardano valued far more the scholarly tributes that were reaching him.

For support of his fair-sized and by no means undemanding household he used money won at gaming—mainly from a Milanese nobleman, Antonio Vimercati by name, who had far more money than sense and would willingly have paid out

4—DC • •

fabulous sums to play at dice with Cardano, whose company he enjoyed for what seem to his Victorian biographer, Professor Fletcher, unmentionable reasons. Unmentionable, that is, except in Latin. Fletcher writes of Vimercati as wearing *quasi vir braccatus*; and the only detectable point of this euphemism seems to be that the wealthy patrician wore a garment "in the semblance of a man's trousers" because he was a homosexual. Or perhaps—even more unspeakable—a Lesbian fetishist? It is unnecessary to probe the mystery. The point is, that Cardano played dice with him daily but won from him only a *real* or two at each game, refusing to accept the crazy bets that Vimercati wanted to place. "I could not have justified my warning in The Book on Games of Chance, that if a person be renowned by noble birth or civil honour it is all the worse for him to play, had I met his wagers. For he was the stupidest man at calculating his chances that ever faced me".[10] Cardano's consideration, however, justifiably allowed him to win a total of two or three gold crowns a day without a pricking of his conscience. On that steady income, and the fees that he earned from his medical practice and lectureships, he managed reasonably well. His improvidence, however, was as great as his father's, and he squandered a great deal of money on the entertainment of "drunken, gluttonous, impudent, unsettled, and lustful musicians" simply for the pleasure of hearing their songs and joining with them in consorts of viols and recorders. He despised their morals but loved their talents, and rarely saw that his fecklessness matched theirs.

Morally dubious though his companions were, the College of Physicians could no longer support any overt antagonism toward him. In 1541 they made him their Rector—an appointment that added to his fame and stature but again brought no money, though by now the royalties for the arithmetic book were beginning to come in—but, as for all authors, not fast enough. Characteristically, he spent much of his time in revising his writings before he sent them to Petreius for printing rather than in embarking on new books. Virtually supported as he was by his gains from Vimercati, he let the wheels of the creative side of his industry turn slower and paid a great deal of attention to more intensive study of the Greek language. But suddenly, at the end of August 1542, Vimercati, overcome by remorse after being given a severe drubbing for his wild ways by a priest of unbending moral rectitude, forswore all his vices including gambling and decided to give the bulk of his wealth to the church. Again Cardano had no cause for complaint, but he remarked wryly, "There was in truth no sign of the bishoprics being void in their coffers; but my own money bag was now of a sudden empty and I was forced to borrow—though those who had most justification for hearing my pleas were most deaf to my needs. Only Fate, brooding darkly in the shadows, was preparing for me cause for another need—not of gold but of fortitude."[11]

IO

1543

It was Tartaglia who assumed the corporeal presence of fate brooding darkly in the shadows. The rival mathematician's resentment at Cardano's independent discovery of the formula he had thought undiscoverable by any brain but his own was aroused again by the publication of *The Practice of Arithmetic* before his own book had been copyrighted. In spite of the fact that Cardano had acknowledged him as prior discoverer he at once published an accusation of plagiarism. Such a charge was untenable and presumably he was told so, for no legal action was fought on the issue. But he continued to brood on the imagined theft and never failed to make disparaging remarks about Cardano in his public lectures.

This man Nicolo Tartaglia, who was to become Cardano's bitterest enemy was born a year before him, in 1500, and inherited no family name, for his father, a tiny fellow called Micheletto the Postman, was the product of a waifs' home and his parents had never been known. He may well have been the bastard of a union between a whore and some drunken reveller. He was abandoned in a hay wagon and taken into the care of some nuns in Brescia and given a rudimentary upbringing until he was old enough to take service as a scullion in the kitchen of a local dignitary. He progressed from the scullery to the stable and eventually acquired a horse of his own with which he took on the postal work between Brescia, Verona, and Bergamo. He met his wife, Maria, a serving girl, when delivering letters to the house of a nobleman in Verona and married her in 1496, bringing her no name but the diminutive of the Michele the nuns had given him, and nothing whatever as a dowry except the casual fees he was given for his postal services. They were,

however, very happy for a short time and had three children, of
whom Nicolo was the second. The marriage was ended by the
death of Micheletto in 1506, when he was ambushed while
crossing the Brescian stretch of the plain lying in the foothills of
the Lombardy Alps. His murderer was a spy in the pay of the
French general Gaston de Foix, who suspected—rightly—the
beginnings of a Brescian uprising against foreign domination
and had ordered the interception of letters that might reveal
embryonic plans. In the particular case of the ambushing and
murder of Micheletto he gained nothing, for the postman's
pouches held only routine correspondence; but he had brought
to widowhood the blameless Maria, who was now left in direst
poverty with three young children whom she could scarcely
feed, let alone educate. But the wretched family managed to
survive while all around them the Brescians' discontent grew
until in 1512 it fermented into open rebellion and the French
were driven from the city. Gaston de Foix, humiliated by having his garrison turned out "by a handful of silkweavers and
armourers", swore bitter revenge. He sacked the city with an
army big enough to subdue a nation and for seven days mercilessly slaughtered the population until forty-six thousand of them
lay amid the smoke and blood of rapine, while the triumphant howling of the bestial victors sounded day and night in
licentious revelry. During that ghastly week hundreds of women
and children streamed into the cathedral seeking refuge, among
them Maria and her three children. But sanctuary was not to be
found even there. A posse of troops set about them solely for the
pleasure of seeing more blood flow and among those who
received sword blows was the child Nicolo. His face was cleft by
a sword through the lips and palate and his injury lost him his
teeth and his power of speech. He was nursed back to health by
the devoted Maria, who was unable to afford any surgeon's fees
or medicaments but so carefully and frequently bathed and
bound the frightful wound that in a few months the boy had
made a scarred recovery—though he was hideous to look upon
and remained so until he was able to grow a beard and hide his
disfigurement. But he was never able to speak properly because
of the damage to his palate, and therefore was called by his
companions "Tartaglia", the stutterer. Because of his mother's

continued poverty he had no schooling and was entirely self taught until, as a young man, he found a patron who sent him to study at Padua, from which seminary he emerged with high honours and a character vain, malicious, and aggrieved—which, considering the misfortune of his early life, was perhaps understandable. Such was the man who now waited to wreak an unwarrantable revenge on Cardano. But the time was not quite ripe.

By 1535 Milan had gradually fallen from its former importance as the capital of northern Italy to an impotent fragment of a dismembered and captive land dominated by Spain. The repeated attempts of France to aid Italy in overthrowing her Spanish conquerors were all unsuccessful—sometimes because of the weakening effects of internecine strife of which the uprising in Brescia in 1512 was typical, sometimes because of the loss of Italian focal power brought about by the ending of the great ducal dynasties. The last Duke of Milan, for instance, had settled his dukedom into the hands of the Emperor Charles V, who rode into the city in triumph in 1533, bringing with him a brief period of prosperity, and a year later the Duke, now a mere minion under the heel of Charles, brought a pale revival of ducal ceremony when he received his sixteen-year-old bride, Cristina of Sweden. "The young princess, whose countenance was more divine than human, rode in under a golden baldaquin, surrounded by twelve of the noblest gentlemen of the city, so splendidly arrayed that each appeared an emperor, and with such great white plumes in their caps that her Excellency seemed to move in the midst of a forest".[1] This brief splendour soon gave way to the gloom of the Milanese when they learnt that the divinely beautiful Cristina had to be supported by a special tax. However, the bridal feast was followed quickly by a more lugubrious pageant, for the Duke died toward the end of 1535 and only one more Sforza, Gian Paolo, was left—bereft of his dukedom and with only the lesser rights of a nobleman left to him. Fanning with his determination a spark of the old Sforza ambitions, he at once set out for Rome to press the pope to support his clam to the dukedom. But on the way he died of a mysterious illness which probably was caused by poison

administered by the emperor's hirelings. Thus the ducal magnificence of the Visconti and Sforza dynasties, which had
invested medieval Milan with horror and beauty, learning and
passion, ended in squalid murder at a roadside tavern.

The efforts of France to oust the Spanish and German occupants from Italy were far from disinterested. Ever since the
treaties of Cambrai and Barcelona were signed by Francis I in
1529, and French claim to Milan was renounced with his signa-
ture, there had been bitter feeling in the French court at the
rising domination of the Austro-Spanish Habsburgs—a bitterness that found its centre in the rivalry between Francis I and
Charles V, begun when Francis had to sign the humiliating
peace after the battle of Pavia in 1525. But though territorially
self-interested and on occasions such as the sack of Brescia wickedly cruel, the French were also concerned to rejuvenate their
flagging inspirations in the arts and sciences by study of the
peaks of Renaissance achievements in Italy. They had the wit to
recognize that an agglomeration of genius represented by such
men as Leonardo, Raphael, Michelangelo, Ariosto, and Machia-
velli was a phenomenon to be exploited by nations less well
favoured; and Francis anticipated by many years the cultural
policy of Louis XIV by treating with special favour all creative
artists and thinkers. Indeed, to him is due the spread of Renaissance influences to France earlier than to the rest of Europe.

It was against a background of political dissolution and military ferment, then, that in 1543 the university of Pavia was
forced to close its doors while soldiers skirmished on its very
doorstep and the simple absence of students forced an economic
stricture that could not be cured without moving to a less
disturbed area. Milan was the nearest and most obvious place to
go to, and early in the spring temporary premises were estab-
ished in the great library that was part of the Augustinian
priory. Once again now Cardano was offered the chair of medicine. The salary was small and there was in any case considerable doubt as to whether it would ever be paid, for the university's treasury was empty; but the professorship carried prestige
and, now that the premises were at the very gates of Milan, the
duties entailed no travelling. And as Rector of the College of

Physicians and Professor of Medicine to a distinguished if econ-
omically shabby university, his medical practice could scarcely
fail to be enhanced. So this time he accepted the offer.

Indifferent though Cardano was to outward appearances,
Lucia had loftier ideas and forced on him the expenses of a
household he could ill afford. He remembered the arguments he
had had with Bandarini over Lucia's support; but he did not
reproach her for her extravagance by reminding her that she
had been willing enough to live with him in poverty when she
married him. "It is marked of women", he wrote, "that their
ambitions cannot expand beyond the social, the regions of their
minds are not of a quality above the trivial".[2] They did not
quarrel. It was understood between them that he should have
his cats, dogs, mules and birds as his companions about the
house; and that she should have a carriage and a servant of her
own as well as the staff who did the ordinary domestic work,
and that she should entertain friends of a more gracious order
than the spirited but vulgar musicians and gamblers who came
for her husband's pleasure. For himself, he walked everywhere,
just as his father had done before him, wrapped in a simple
cloak and with a mule carrying his books, for he would not
inflict on Giovanni, now nine years old, the indignity of being a
beast of burden as he himself had been to Fazio. He was only
just past forty, but his mien was professorial, his back bent, his
walk eccentric in the variation of its speed, his speech unpredict-
ably explosive and irascible, his manner in general with his
patients gentle and with his students severe; but if called to
minister to rich men pained by indigestion caused by gross
indulgence, or questioned by students showing uncommon per-
ception, then severity went to the patients and gentleness to the
students. He had, we are told by the bitter Tartaglia, "a loud
laugh like the bray of an ass and a mind empty of all but great
plains of ignorance".[3] But that was merely the feeble invective
of an enemy impotently grinding his teeth in the outward
expression of insult while an abrasive malice did its work within.

On 25 May 1543 Cardano's second son, to be christened
Aldo, was born—"A fine child with no disfigurement or fault
attending him, or any trouble to my wife". And on the night of

the same date he had one of his visionary dreams in which he was bidden by "An awful figure sitting among rolling clouds to parallel the work of my loins with the work of my mind and bring forth a new book". He took this command to mean that a *magnum opus* should be completed before his supposed approaching death and immediately on waking he began to plan his *Ars Magna*, a definitive work on the great art of arithmetic, a work for scholars rather than the populace, and the book whereby Tartaglia was to engineer his revenge—though Cardano naturally knew nothing of that, and even if he had would not have damped down his feverish activity upon it. His activity was in fact so concentrated that he had to be told by the serving woman that patients needed his attention. Even then he sometimes disdained to answer their calls. That should have earned him reprimands from the College of Physicians, which in theory was all things ethical if in practice it was hidebound and smug; but he was himself Rector and therefore escaped such consequences. There is no indication that the calls he refused to answer were any but the most trivial; but the evidence of their existence was accreting in the devilishly meticulous annals recorded by Tartaglia. And they would be recalled at precisely the right moment.

The rest of that year, 1543, was marked by his ceaseless industry on the *Ars Magna* and increasing debts caused by the loss of income from Vimercati. Typically, he allowed the debts to accumulate while his own patients remained indebted to him—either through his forgetfulness or their inability to pay. When a proportion of his salary from the university was paid (it amounted to one hundred gold crowns, less than half the due sum) it was immediately swallowed up by interest due to moneylenders, who were all too eager to continue to advance him capital sums secured by his house and the respectability of his position, or by expectations from Fazio's inheritance, which was still enmeshed in endless legal squabbles. He is not enlightening about the social consequences of his poverty. Did he have to insist that Lucia should contribute to stringent economic measures by lowering her social sights? It seems doubtful. He prob-ably ignored the whole thing and allowed the debts to mount.

He was the sort of man who could have been persuaded to sign anything that would stop people bothering him for money he didn't at the moment possess, or, within his own household, to agree to anything that would give him peace and quiet. Such men are often said to excuse themselves from the practical responsibilities of life by conveniently assuming an other-worldly concern for more cerebral matters. But with Cardano it was not a matter of convenience but of necessity. He was in the midst of a period of great creative activity which, amid the seething cauldron of destructive influences overturned by political and religious megalomaniacs and spreading through southern Europe with apocalyptic force, was reflected as bravely and weakly as a tiny star.

It will not be out of place to look briefly at the molten forces that ran like fiery rivers through the continent.

The despotic rule of the Emperor Charles V is at its apogee. He has extended his Habsburg grip to embrace the Netherlands, Spain, and Milan; he has encircled France and says he dreams of an harmonious Christendom that will hold fast against the menace of Turkey. Erasmus of Rotterdam, architect of the Reformation, is proving himself to be an inadequate quietist steeped in moderation and lacking entirely the fiery spirit of Luther, as his own supine words prove: "Let others affect martyrdom; for myself I am unworthy of the honour". The cruelties and excesses of the Roman church, diminished by reforming zeal, suddenly flare again, ignited by the Luciferine spark of the Counter-reformation. The revenue for the extravagances of the papal court is found from the sale of pardons for every imaginable and unimaginable sin, "even the rape of God's mother, if that were possible". The Holy Father extends his benevolence to the promise of eternal life in paradise upon payment of the appropriate fee. There are written and promulgated edicts that ensure the great commercial success of the traffic in pardons. Heresy is the greatest of the crimes against the church because it attacks where she is weakest: in her assumption of temporal power and the consequent corruption. But even heretics can buy themselves off by oiling the wheels of repentance with the grease of bribery. Firm heretics, however, are rarely repentant. For them, the inquisition and the *auto-da-fé* offer a suitable punishment and at the same time a public spectacle. No money to purchase a papal bull being forthcoming, heretics are flung into a dungeon where they may languish for a short or long time as the personal cruelty of the priest or monk making the accusation may dictate. Now, not even money can affect the decision. The victim is taken to the torture chamber and the black-robed operator of every conceivable apparatus for the infliction of pain awaits him. In the light of flaming torches he is stripped naked while the screw, the rack, the flame, the red-hot pincers, are made ready. Only confession can end the tortures; but the informing priests, whose idea of propagating the faith they represent seems somewhat different from Christ's, have been disappointed of their fiscal dues, and the victims' confessions now can lead only to the stake. Bodily broken to the point of death they are now clothed in yellow robes embroidered with devils, paper mitres, and gags. (The gags are symbolic only : the victims' tongues have already been ripped from their throats to prevent them ever again from uttering heretical words.) In the public square where the people crowd, lusting for excitement, the magistrates, nobility, and clergy form ranks behind whom are ranged on caparisoned horses the gorgeously attired inquisitors who have conducted the "trial" of the victims. The bishop preaches on the evils of heresy and the justice of the inquisition. The fifty-first psalm is sung by the whole throng while the fire at the base of the scaffold is lit. Stake after burning stake is thrust into the heart of the flames, with the victims' bodies bound thereto—those who have found the strength to repent of their heresy being strangled first to the accompaniment of the triumphal yells of the crowd. The spectacle continues as long as there is flesh to burn; and at the end of the *auto-da-fé* everyone crowds into the cathedral to worship.

Imperial edicts are issued by the Emperor to suppress the Reformation in the Netherlands, whence Erasmus came. Charles has no power of suzerain in Germany, which is not part of his heritage; but Luther is branded all the same as "a devil clothed in the form of a man, clothed in the dress of a priest the better to bring the human race to death and damnation", and his disciples and converts are to be punished by death and forfeiture of goods. Spain has the immense empire of newly discovered America added to her already vast dominions in Austria, Africa, the Netherlands, Italy, and France. Charles aggravates discontent by his foreign birth, high taxes, the robbing of the country of its gold, and the sale of privileged posts to foreigners. Revolts and civil war are the outcome, but Charles allies himself with Henry VIII of England and invades that part of France that is not already subdued by his minions. Then, as his power grows, until at the age of thirty he is conqueror of most of Europe and much of north Africa, Spain too is completely subjugated. In Germany and Switzerland the radical group of extreme Lutherans, the Anabaptists, swells in size, reforming zeal, and contagious madness until they form an armed insurrection that captures the city of Münster and are defeated only when the Bishop captures their leader, the so-called "King of Sion" and has him pinched to death with red-hot tongs. The Anabaptists' intensity also takes on a crazed form that causes them to strip naked in bitter weather and run madly through the streets shrieking, "Woe! Woe! The wrath of God!" When arrested they refuse to put on clothes but merely observe, with some justification, "We are the naked truth".[4]

In the midst of the cacophony compounded from the crack of shot, the swish of the sword, the singing of holy mass, the crackling of flames, the screams of victims, and the muttering of prayers, there is still one force that can halt the advance of troops and send the generals back from their reconnaissances filled with doubts : disease. Small-pox and bubonic plague are the endemic killers and they can sweep through a city in days with more effect than can an army of mercenaries. Also, there is what is for many a mysterious new disease that has manifested itself in epidemic proportions since Columbus's return from Haiti* in 1493 and is called euphemistically "the Spanish disease". This was spread by Columbus's sailors to the mercenary troops in Barcelona and Seville and by them to the French force that had invested Naples in the same year. Cosmopolitan in their allegiances and peripatetic in their movements these soldiers, and the women they used, were of course the most cer-

---

* Which he of course called Española.

tain instruments of infection; and syphilis too took its grip on
Europe. By 1540 that grip had become ferocious and neither
cause nor cure had been found.

Such, shown in a compact but necessarily over-simplified
sketch, was the condition of the continent when Doctor Cardano entered upon the greatest creative period of his career.

II

1544-1545

As with so many men whose achievements indicate a fury of
activity, Cardano appears from his journals to have lived each
day without haste or fuss except for occasional impetuous outbursts against students, patients, or servants. He never rose till
two hours after sunrise; he then had a light breakfast of raisins,
water, and bread, and settled down in his workroom with his
cats, dogs, goats and birds surrounding him. He worked with his
feet naked in spite of their continual coldness, believing that
exercise was better than shoes and that it was also good for the
brain to change its course of thought frequently; so at irregular
intervals he would stop writing and walk twenty or so times
round his table while his mind switched itself to another subject
or his wife or children wandered into the room to be conversed
with or engaged awhile with games and riddles. A student
would be on hand to help him with his researches, fill his costly
inkstand and lay his paper in the way he approved. Patients
would arrive or have to be visited, lectures must be prepared
and delivered, consultations with other doctors, philosophers,
and mathematicians must be arranged. His midday meal—an
eggyolk mixed with wine, and a slice of bread—he would take
without stopping work; but if one of his musician friends was
about he would listen to one or two songs while he jotted down
ideas for "machines and devices"—ideas that came to him most
easily when there was music in the air. In the evening in suitable weather he liked to fish for an hour, again with a student
or his eldest son at hand to write down thoughts or notions that
occurred to him; and he would then take his late meal of veal,
shellfish, carp, gudgeon, or salted herrings, followed by fruit and
onions spiced with rue and wormwood. ("Five things may be

taken freely by all save old men", he observed marginally in a manuscript on morals. "They are bread, fish, cheese, wine, and water. And four things are to be taken moderately, and they are meat, eggs, raisins, and oil. Saffron and salt must be condiments, and mastix and corriander are for medicine".) His evening meal over, he would play at dice, chess, or cards, or listen to more music; then, late at night, return to his workroom and revise the day's writings or consider his appearance and health.

So far as his appearance was concerned, he disliked his own face and kept a hand mirror by him as if childishly to confirm from time to time that there had been no improvement. His beard concealed the plague-warts on his cheeks and chin, and he kept his cap pulled down over the one on his forehead; but the largest was on his nose, and was, he says, "as repulsive as a gaping wound or a condition of the pox". He was indifferent to clothes and made the few he had serve him for years. They were old-fashioned and ignored altogether the Spanish influence that tended toward jewelled magnificence. "I care little for the garb of prosperity", he wrote, "but my extravagance for books and fine writing materials is with me like a lust".

As for his health, at this time when according to the predictions of the stars his life was approaching its end, he gloomily acquired new aches and pains daily to reinforce his conviction that the stars must be proved right. "My flesh has been tainted from the first with evil humours", he notes with characteristic self-pity in June 1544, and now to my burdens is added the gout". Clearly most of his ailments were imaginary or unsevere, for he scarcely ever records that he has to take to his bed because of them. Perhaps he saw himself as a stoic enduring the ills of the flesh without complaint. More probably, there was an ambivalence in his nature that allowed him to view his hypochondria with slightly cynical detachment.

His day's work done, he "entered into new worlds of trouble or perplexity in sleep". He recalled his dreams with remarkable clarity and sought meanings and warnings in all of them. His dead mother appeared to him "wearing the scarlet dress she used to wear when occupied in work about the house". She

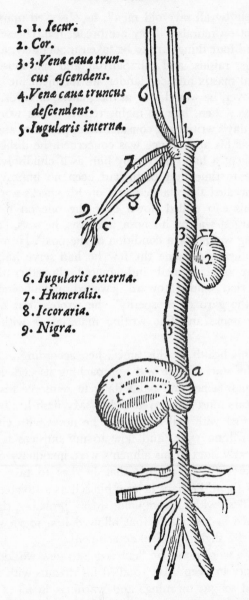

1. 1. *Iecur.*
2. *Cor.*
3. 3. *Vena caua truncus aſcendens.*
4. *Vena caua truncus deſcendens.*
5. *Iugularis interna.*

6. *Iugularis externa.*
7. *Humeralis.*
8. *Iecoraria.*
9. *Nigra.*

The circulation of the blood as supposed by Cardano

summoned him to join her next year and he saw this as confirmation that the stars were right in their prophecy; and indeed a year hence (in 1545) he narrowly escaped death when his mule, whose halter he had fastened to his belt, took fright and dragged him into the path of a wagon which only just missed crushing his body. He dreamed one night of Alexander the Great, Hephaestion, and a lion, and saw there the symbolism of his overcoming of adversity. He was forever receiving reminders, admonitions, and directions in the form of elaborate visionary playacting; and in nearly all these dream scenas death hovered patiently. And indeed, consequently or not, death was not far off—but not for him.

In medicine his achievements were often remarkable and seldom less than noteworthy. The construction of the human body was still not understood with certainty. Artists like Leonardo, Michelangelo, and Dürer had by their studies of the body considerably advanced the knowledge of anatomy; but the circulatory system was not understood; no-one had investigated the theory of infection; such surgical instruments as there were were crude; the microscope had not been invented; the atomic construction of matter had not been dreamed of; embryology, neurology, and epidemiology were fields of learning far beyond the horizon. Cardano's achievements did not lie in the contemporary advancement of any of these branches of medicine but in his ability to effect cures as it were instinctively, basing his treatments on what we should now call common sense. One such cure had much to do with the subsequent history of venereology.

His printer friend Ottaviano Scoto had caught some disease that was causing putrefaction and shrinkage of his genitals. So little was known about the venereal diseases in the sixteenth century that they were often confused with leprosy. Gonorrhoea, unknown by that name but established since time immemorial was called "the burning disease". Syphilis, though comparatively rare until Columbus's return from America in 1493, was thought to be a developed form of "the burning disease" because it too was characterized by sores, discharges, and pain associated with the genital organs, though in its later stages it resulted in rotting of the facial flesh, which gonorrhoea did not.

That rotting and the consequent revolting effects, plain for all to
see, earned it the name of "the wicked disease" (*nefandum
infirmitatum*), as well as "the Spanish disease", since it revealed
the supposed promiscuity of the sufferer's life. Both John of
Gaunt and Pope Ubertinus VIII had died of it in the Middle
Ages; but the Renaissance and Reformation, one of the great
epochs of promiscuity, threw between history's colonnades a
greater number of famous victims than could be found in the
previous thousand years. Benvenuto Cellini, Philip II of Spain,
Henry VIII, Ivan the Terrible, and Mary Tudor were among
them. By the end of the sixteenth century Europe was so
scourged by the disease that the fashion of euphemizing or
localizing it by the adjective "Spanish" had died out. It had
become simply "the great pox". Licentiousness was so much a
characteristic of the age that "the wicked disease" had become
no more than a smirking reference used by the coy.

Scoto, artisan though he was, placed the customary faith in
sorcery and had visited a supposed wise man who had recom-
mended the sucking of the sores by a beggar, poulticing with a
live bisected frog, and immersion of the affected parts in the
disembowelled body of a mule. That treatment proving ineffective he had gone to his friend Cardano. "This affliction of the
pudenda", the doctor wrote, "is clearly the same as that which
mortified the parts of Caesar Borgia and is written of in a
treatise by his physician Gaspare Torella, who calls it *Pudenda-
grum sen Morbum Gallicum*. We think of this thing that it is but
an advancement of the burning disease that all know of, so
widely is it spread throughout the world and a heritage only of
uneasy [he means unclean] living. But the discharge that comes
from that is not as Scoto's. I have seen too much for me not to
know. Here in this greater pox is work for me that it may be
cured". Work indeed. How he arrived at the proper treatment—
or what he thought was proper treatment—he does not reveal.
Possibly by guesswork or by having read in medical literature of
the "Saracen Ointment" used by the Crusaders. His antidote,
however, he gives in recipe: it is a compound of animal fat,
charcoal, bayleaves, oil of scorpions, and mercury. The mercury,
he notes, has been tried before for "the burning disease" and
has proved ineffective. Whether he hoped to prove that

"the greater pox" was entirely different from the older disease, though also venereal in origin, he does not say. But Scoto's sores and discharges reacted favourably to the ointment after some six months. This in itself is not remarkable: mercury is indeed an antidote to syphilis, and even today, with Salvarsan, penicillin, iodides and the sulpha drugs leading the field in its treatment, is still used. What is remarkable is that he offered evidence that more than three hundred years later led Philippe Ricord, a French doctor researching in venereal diseases, to establish finally that the organisms causing gonorrhoea and syphilis are quite different. "It was chance that led me to Cardano's works in the Library", Ricord says in the preface to the paper on venereology that lays the proof before the medical world, "and there is no doctor before or since who so convinced me that we must make of this infection *two* infections and look for their causes separately". In that one branch of medicine alone, then, Cardano's intuition may be said to have made a positive contribution. We have already seen how in his treatment of tuberculosis he intuitively experimented with the healing qualities of clear country air and rest and established the principle of the sanatorium. In later pages his method of treating a notable personage for another "incurable" disease, asthma, will be given some attention; for it was by way of that association with so influential a patient that he found riches strewn at his feet and fame glowing round him like the incandescence of one of his dreams.

But Cardano's working day of seemingly leisurely tempo was by no means limited to practice and study of medicine. The "machines and devices" that he tells us were inspired by music were sketched on many manuscript sheets that, like Leonardo's, often delineate several stages of thought and development in invention. Leonardo's working drawings were of course beautiful in themselves; Cardano's were never that, for he had no talent in draughtsmanship and his drawings were extremely crude and had to be re-done by others—not always displaying much more talent than his own—before they found their way into his books of popular science.

One of his inventions at this time was evidently the result of

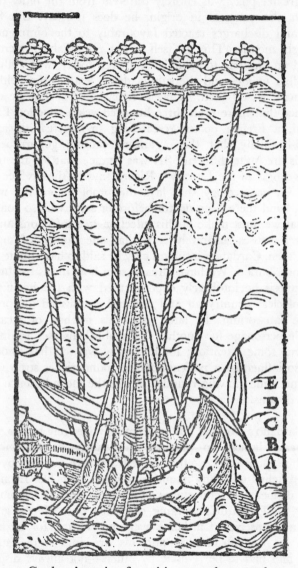

Cardano's notion for raising a sunken vessel

his recalling to mind his visit to Venice with Fazio in 1515, when he saw one of the Flanders galleys sunk in the harbour there by a mutinous crew. It was a method of raising a sunken vessel by attaching to it a series of ropes that were fastened at their upper ends to small heavily ballasted boats lying low in the water by reason of the weight of the ballast. As the ballast was jettisoned, so the buoyancy of the boats allowed them to rise in the water, raising with them the sunken vessel sufficiently for it to be moved to a shallower spot. This and many other inventions of Cardano's fertile brain may be said to exhibit a complex logic similar to that shown in the joyful lunacies of that twen-

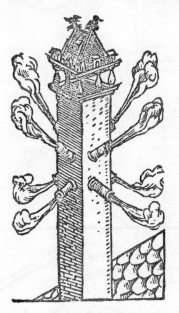

Cardano's method of smoke extrusion left space for a dovecote on top of the chimney

tieth century genius the late Heath Robinson; but, as with Mr Robinson's "inventions", it could be demonstrated that they worked. Also belonging to this inventive period is a quaint method of smoke extrusion to prevent down-draught making the smoke billow out into the room. Cardano's notion was to close the top of the chimney stack with an ornamental dovecote and to extrude the smoke instead through a number of small chimney pots protruding at different angles through the sides of the

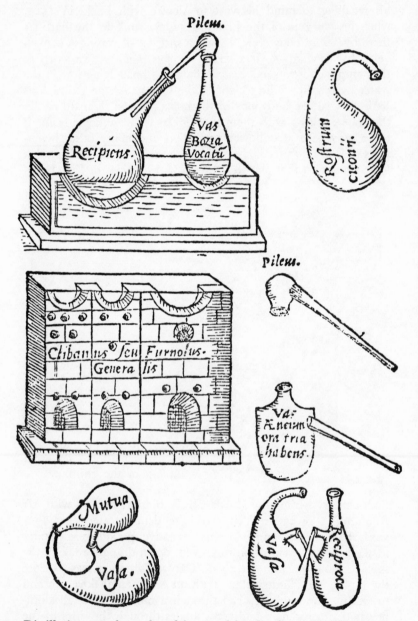

Distillation vessels used and invented by Cardano. The furnace is also his invention

stack. By increasing the number of orifices over which air currents flowed the smoke was naturally carried away quicker. Devices that have become familiar as everyday gadgets in the twentieth century are to be found in *De Subtilitate Rerum* and *De Rerum Varietate*, his two books on popular science for which he was busily, in 1544 and 1545, recording the material. Since he rarely found, or indeed troubled to look for, smiths, armourers, architects, or horologists who could transform his notions into practical shape, they were usually copied or re-invented in later days by those with minds more interested in the pecuniary advantages of pressing upon the world the machinery needed to keep pace with the advancement of learning; for surely enough, in accordance with the present-day Mr Parkinson's law, so soon as a theory had been unravelled from

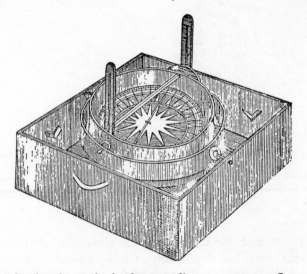

Cardano's method of suspending a compass. It was an adaptation of this idea that resulted in the universal ʲoint and the Cardan shaft of the motor-car

the knotty mysteries of the universe, so some way of adapting it to the advantage, supposed or real, of civilization had to be discovered. There are to be found in Cardano's notebooks

designs for a pressure lamp exactly similar to the Tilley lamp
used today; a clock escapement using an oscillating weight;
many original ideas for retorts and distilling vessels; a system of
shorthand; a compass with its needle suspended in alcohol; a
combination lock precisely similar in principle to those used on
modern safes; and of course the universal joint for transmitting
mechanical energy through an angle that alone of his inventions
bears his name today. The Cardan shaft that connects the gear-
box of the motor-car to the rear wheels and allows the flexibility

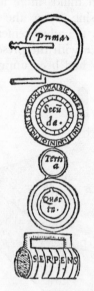

Cardano's forerunner
of the modern com-
bination lock. Only
the keyword—in this
case "*Serpens*"—would
permit the cogs to turn
and raise the wards of
the lock

needed to absorb the varying vertical movement of the sprung
rear axle uses his ingeniously simple universal joint—two
U-shaped links fixed to the ends of the shafts to be joined and
coupled by being pivoted to the periphery of an intervening
disc. Originally this was invented by Cardano to permit the
angular driving of a multiple Archimedes screw. (The multiple
screw also was his invention and was intended to raise water
from low-lying streams to irrigate hillside fields.) But he had
realized a need for a flexible axle as he followed the baldachin
of Charles V when the Emperor entered Milan in 1533 and

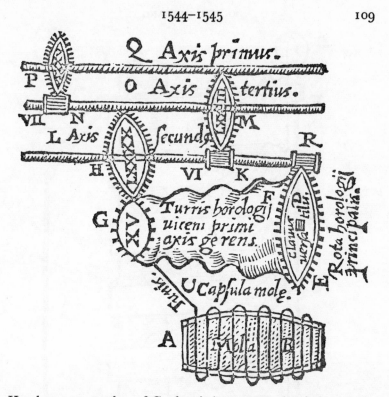

Horology was another of Cardano's interests: a sketch for an improved clockwork mechanism

saw how the wheeled litter absorbed through its frame every bump in the ill-made roads. "For an Emperor, however foreign to Milan he may be, to be disturbed and tumbled in his riding is so far without dignity that people may laugh and incur the royal displeasure", he wrote with concern at that time. More than ten years passed, however, before he thought of the flexible joint; and another three before, in 1548, he saw how it could be used in the undercarriage of a royal vehicle. By which time his fame and social position were so much advanced that he was able to arrange for the court armourers and wheelwrights to adapt the device for use in the Emperor's baldachin.

In mathematics as in all other fields of activity he made great

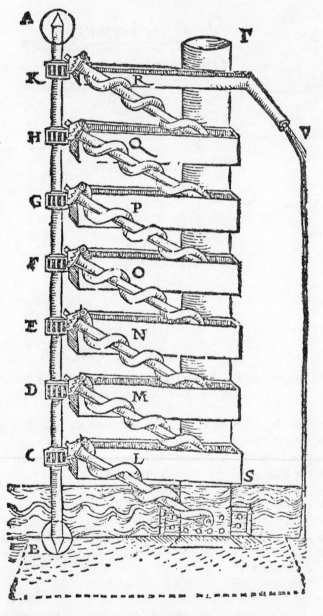

The multiple Archimedes screw invented by Cardano

advances during these years when he expected death to come upon him every day. His *Ars Magna* approached—and, in 1545, achieved—completion. In it he explained the whole theory of cubic equation, which explanation had a far-reaching effect on the work of all the great mathematicians who were to follow him. And with its publication the smouldering enmity between him and Tartaglia burst into flame. "Every step for-

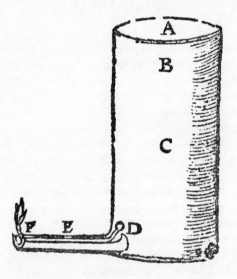

Cardano's oil lamp gave a steadier
light because the oil was kept in the
container by vacuum

ward is to be halted by some matching trouble", he was to write years later; "and every joy is to be matched with a sorrow. And so as I was known to fame and fortune, neither was I neglected by adversity".

I2

1546-1551

Indeed adversity did not neglect him. Sometimes its machinations were bizarre. One night he and Lucia and the three children went to bed—"under one cover, in our custom"—and in
the early hours were awakened by a great trembling of the
house. The house, though grand, was already old when Chiara
bought it, and it had been neglected and now gave up its
strength completely—the rear wall falling out into the courtyard
leaving the rooms exposed like a doll's house and sending great
clouds of choking dust down upon the occupants. The servants
fled, the animals bristled and bellowed with alarm, and the bed
holding the master of the house and his family collapsed with its
occupants frantically clawing at each other and coughing and
sneezing as the dust fell upon them. Excepting Aldo, the baby,
they were wearing only nightcaps.[1]

No one was hurt in this farcical occurrence, but it decided
Cardano to reverse a decision he had just made. The tide of war
having retreated from Pavia the syndics of the university had
determined to move back there from Milan and had asked
Cardano to continue in his professorship of medicine at the
same salary—two hundred and forty crowns. Remarking drily
that the salary was low by the accepted standards even if he
received all of it, which frequently he didn't, Cardano had
thanked the syndics for their offer and refused it. He had, he
said, a mountain of work to be climbed in Milan and preferred
to remain there and tackle it. Now, however, with his house
fallen about his ears he was forced to move. Characteristically,
he took the incident to be an omen of his own doom—"Such
omens often come triply, and this surely is the first"—and
accepted it with resignation. But unlike the man in the oriental

tale who fled from Death after an encounter in the market place only to find the grinning figure waiting by appointment in Samarra, he did not think to escape. The move back to Pavia was simply a matter of convenience. "Death will find me there as readily as here", he notes; "but with my wife unwell it is greatly more convenient to move to apartments adjunctive to my duties in the academy than to search for and buy a house here in Milan".[2]

That is the first of surprisingly few references to Lucia's declining health. He is never explicit about the cause, or even the symptoms. Possibly the irony of finding himself successful in curing so many of his patients but unable to cure his own wife made him reluctant to record the course of her illness. Morley in his *Life of Cardano* says she was "perhaps worn down by the succession of anxieties"; but although it is true that in the early days of their marriage she suffered homelessness, starvation, and the loss of the jewellery and finery that had been her only dowry, she had for some time been sharing her husband's fame and modest fortune, and had indeed reverted to the social standing that had been her lot before marriage and had spent much of his income and hastened him by her extravagances toward the parlous financial state that he was to flounder in for some time yet—though he remained as indifferent to its effects as ever before. Also, she was still a young woman—she was thirty-three—and the few years of penury had been passed when she was even younger and fresher from the relatively luxurious surroundings of her father's home. So it seems improbable that she was worn down by anxieties. Some organic disease seems much more likely. Since Cardano mentions only such vague terms as "decline", "paleness", "lassitude", "choler", and the like one can hardly speculate on what disease she suffered from; and she must fade from the scene with as little ceremony as Cardano marks her going. He does not even specify the date of her death, but it was certainly toward the end of 1546. Up to that time there are only vague references to her illness. After her death he wrote, "The occupations of my workroom were previously necessary to moderate my love for my wife and children. Now only my children need me and my occupations may be increased.... She [Lucia] was brave, indomitable in spirit, gentle, affectionate, fine to look upon". Her social extravagances were evidently of little account to him. There is a pathos in the brief list of her sterling qualities. And indeed their number is greater than may be found in many a wife. Because of his reluctance or inability to find words to record the course of her illness as he would have recorded that of an ordinary patient, his tenderness glows the more in those few words so briefly summing up his loss. She has been there in his journals but always very much in the background; for, his pleasure in her company being continual, he had no need to convince himself of it in words. Now, in a simple sentence, she takes the foreground, but too late and too shortly to make an impact on the reader of the journals. And indeed that is as it should be, for Cardano expected no readers for his journals and it was only by mistake that some of them reached print.

A widower with no understanding of domestic problems, he now was forced to increase his household. He had undertaken Giovanni's education himself, but the little girl, Chiara, and the baby, Aldo, were outside his scope. He engaged a housekeeper and on her advice took into his house an extra nursemaid and an extra manservant. This was the sort of advice that made for a splendidly comfortable household and a heavy drain on the purse. With no-one but himself to inspect the housekeeping books—and, having inspected them, to nod sagely and agree them—he was the easy victim of every unscrupulous servant who drifted into his employ. Lucia in her wildest extravagances had never approached the expenses which now mounted round him. A mathematician familiar with the most abstruse problems of algebra, he yet was incapable of analysing the arithmetical prevarications of anyone with a mind to deceive him. Robbed right and left, he was forced to yield to the pressures of moneylenders by spending more time than he cared to spend in gambling, since that was the only reasonably sure method known to him of supplementing his income. But lacking a willing victim of the character of the once foolish but now reformed Vimercati, he was forced to neglect much legitimate work in the squalid pursuit of money to be tipped into a bottomless well. Mercifully, his plight was discovered by Lucia's mother, Bandarini's widow, a dominating woman named Thaddaea, who after he had suffered three years of systematic robbery moved in and took charge of the household. As a châtelaine she inspired so much awe that all the servants fled at the very knowledge of her imminent arrival. Cardano was bothered no more with domestic dishonesty. A bond of understanding united him to Thaddaea. Formidably capable, she ran her own household in Sacco and Cardano's in Pavia with equal success, travelling between the two at unpredictable intervals that left the servants in both continually on the *qui vive*. She left him to his work, ensured the tranquillity necessary for him to conduct it, and, if she disapproved of some of his feckless musical and gambling friends, kept her counsel. He treated her with respect and accepted her advice in all domestic concerns.

He had expected death daily and death had come. But curiously he makes no attempt to reconcile with the predictions of his own horoscope the fact that it was Lucia whom death had claimed. He simply writes no more of his own daily expectations of doom. He emphasizes instead the accuracy of his astrological predictions as to his fame. And indeed, horoscope regarded or regardless, during the three years since Lucia's death he had become known internationally, not only through his books, which Petreius and Osiander were continuing to publish, but through the quarrel with Tartaglia, which in these years reached its climax—though not the climax of Tartaglia's vindictiveness—and through his practice as a physician.

Of the quarrel, there is an immense store of evidence, little of which is remarkable for either its wit or its narrative interest. Its origins, as I have explained, lay in the testy exchanges over the publication of *The Practice of Arithmetic* in 1540. Tartaglia having been worsted in that argument and in his attempt to bring an action for plagiarism, nursed his grievance until the publication of the *Ars Magna* in 1545. In that work Cardano naturally made use of the algebraic equations he had thought out for himself when Tartaglia had refused to share the knowledge with him; and again he acknowledged that Tartaglia had discovered the equations first. But this time, by a slip of pen or memory, he wrote that Tartaglia had communicated the discovery to him and given him permission to use it. It may perhaps not have been a slip but a muddled attempt at a generous gesture on Cardano's part. If it was, he reaped nothing but scorn and contumely for it. There was an immediate swingeing attack by Tartaglia denying ever having given Cardano permission and accusing him of theft. Cardano kept silent, presumably thinking that the charge was too ridiculous to answer. But his most brilliant pupil, Lodovico Ferrari, who had come to him as a servant boy and been turned by his tutelage into a brilliant mathematician, took it upon himself to send a scathing reply. Within a few months Tartaglia and Ferrari were publishing cartels in broadsheet form and flinging insults at one another in public controversy. Matters were worsened by the publication, during this time, of Tartaglia's *New Problems and Inventions* which had a hastily added postscript in which he made a great many insulting remarks about Cardano. "In this", Ferrari wrote, "you have the infamy to say that he is ignorant in mathematics, and you call him uncultured and simple minded, a man of low standing and coarse talk and other similar offending words too tedious to repeat. Since His Excellency is prevented by the rank he holds, and because this matter concerns me personally since I am his creature, I have taken it upon myself to make known publicly your deceit and malice". The acid-natured Tartaglia could scarcely be expected to resist making capital out of the phrase "his creature" and did so on every possible occasion, adding always a verbal or visible smirk.

The cartels grew longer and more bitter. They were sold in the streets (which was the custom of the time) and sent to all the leading scholars and noblemen in many cities. They circulated throughout Europe, taking Cardano's name with them; and other scholars entered into the arguments and published broadsheets of their own, taking sides, elaborating the problems in both Cardano's and Tartaglia's books and in effect performing the functions of critics and publicity agents. For eighteen months during 1547 and 1548 the quarrel grew in intensity, the invective became more biting, the challenges more disputatious. Cardano all this time remained unsnared, reaping the benefit of his spreading fame while Ferrari acted as amanuensis, champion, and challenger. Clearly the outcome could only be a public

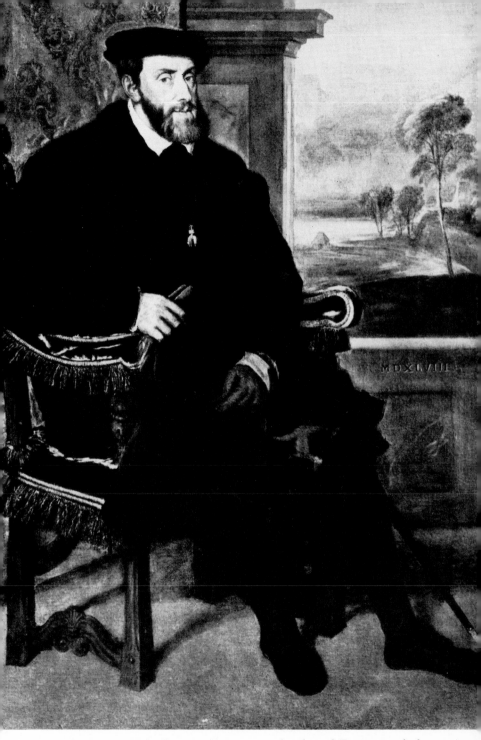

Charles V, Holy Roman Emperor and ruler of Europe and the
New World until his abdication in 1558. From him Cardano
obtained copyright protection for *The Practice of Arithmetic*

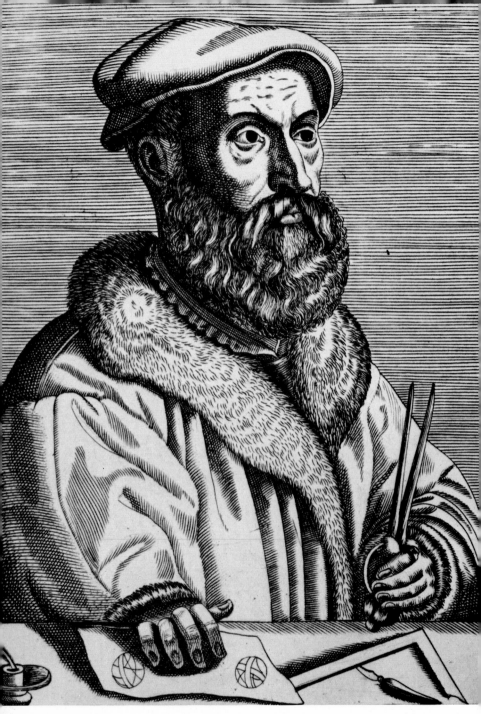

Nicolo Tartaglia, son of a postman, brilliant mathematician and Cardano's brooding, ruthless enemy

contest similar to that between Tartaglia and Fiore, with questions posed in advance and an arbiter appointed to decide the winner. This was arranged and took place on Friday, 10 August 1548, in the garden of the big church of Frati Zoccolanti. The Governor of Milan, Don Ferrante di Gonzaga, was the supreme arbiter and there were present on the dais with him all the distinguished officers, nobles, and scholars of the city. The disputants stood at desks facing each other with canopies over their heads. Behind them on benches rising in tiers were ranged their supporters. On the grass between them were flowers to signify the sweetness of the atmosphere that was supposed to be maintained. In fact the atmosphere was early made extremely sour by Tartaglia, who disadvantaged himself by exceeding his time, introducing irrelevant argument, losing his temper, and turning what should have been an occasion for public entertainment into a rowdy shouting match in which he effectively tore his own scholarly reputation to shreds. Again and again he was urged by the judges and officials to "resume the dignified mantle of the scholar"; but he was apparently incapable of anything but the wildest invective and irresponsibility in dealing with the questions posed by Ferrari, who, whenever he was able to get a word in edgewise, proved himself to be in every way the better scholar. The dispute continued all day and at the end of it Tartaglia through no fault but his own suffered an ignominious defeat and was forced to return, sullen and hateful, to his home in Brescia.[4] One cannot but feel a momentary compassion for this man in whom the seeds of instability had been nourished by childhood environment and had grown into weeds choking the flowers of his own brilliance; but nor can one be entirely surprised that having now a second and much larger grievance to nurse, he should seek his revenge more subtly.

Throughout this great dispute Cardano, the man whom it most concerned and who was the recipient of the fame it conjured from the scholarly attention of all Europe, remained in the background. There is no indication that he even attended the public debate. It was "Cardano's rule" that was the subject, but the youth Ferrari was the protagonist. No doubt Cardano coached his favourite and most brilliant pupil, but his wish was that Ferrari should gain the attention of the world. Which indeed he did. So much attention, in fact, that in due course the Emperor Charles V summoned him to his court and offered him the post of tutor to his son. Ferrari was impulsive and hot-headed and dared to tell the Emperor that he wanted a higher salary than went with the post. With surprising indulgence Charles took this criticism smiling and told Ferrari that he would have him appointed to a more lucrative position—that of tax assessor for Gonzaga, the Governor of Milan. There could scarcely have existed a more profitable post (unless it were that of a priest extorting fees for pardons), and Ferrari remained in it for several years, being forced to leave it only for the ignoble reason that he suffered from a fistula on the buttock which was worsened by riding on horseback—a necessary means of conveyance with such a wide territory to cover. He amassed a great deal of money during his tenure of appointment, however, and was able to transfer to cushioned comfort in the secretarial service of Gonzaga's brother, who was Cardinal of Mantua. He remained throughout his life a staunch friend of Cardano and when the time came for fuel to be heaped on Tartaglia's flaming enmity he was immediately at Cardano's side.

Having succeeded in his attempts to attract the attention of the scholarly world to Ferrari, and at the same time drawn to himself the attention of an even wider audience, Cardano now received offer after offer. He was not of course surprised. "This was the time when my stars were crossed for fortune". Nor was he averse. "Destined for fame, I sought it; visited by it, I exploited it". The name of Doctor Cardano rang through the halls of philosophy, astrology, mathematics, science, and medicine. Books, tracts, and treatises by the score came from the press of Petrieus; for not only were the thirty-four manuscripts advertised in *The Practice of Arithmetic* all published, but they were constantly added to by way of Cardano's phenomenal industry. It is true that some of his works would be considered today little more than articles in terms of length—varying between ten and twenty thousand words—but to turn out fifty or more such in the course of a year, as he did, commands respect. And respect was his. But he had also gripped the public imagination in the branch of learning in which kings, ecclesiastics, and commoners alike were interested : medicine. Learned men

might praise and discuss him in the groves of academe, but
bodily ills were understood by everybody and disease was as
great a foe as despotism. A champion who tourneyed with the
malefic horsemen of pain and decline was a hero to all if he had
proved his worth. And Cardano had done that by effecting
cures that were remarkable rather than numerous. Like that of
every doctor, much of his daily work was routine and could
have been accomplished by any practitioner; but he brought to
the difficult cases an attitude that had little in common with the
mumb-jumbo of sorcery and superstition that was a legacy of
the Middle Ages. Rather, it reverted to the aphoristic teaching
of Hippocrates, Galen, and Maimonides and was aided by the
anatomical revelations of the great artists and his own staunch
refusal to be misled in his diagnoses by mercenary considera-
tions. (Such were the recourse of many doctors of those days :
they would prescribe the most expensive treatment for the simplest troubles, putting themselves in league with the pharmacists
and taking a handsome percentage of the profits for this mutual
assistance.) Often, in fact, his patients had to remind him to
render an account; and even more often he would refuse to do
so when the patients were poor. But he always accepted without
compunction retaining fees from the rich, who groaned at the
rigorousness of the régimes he imposed upon them and enjoyed
their improving health with a kind of inverted masochism. They
would pass his name round among themselves rather as the
names of psychiatrists are circulated today; and the fact that he
treated such fashionable popularity with contempt seemed only
to encourage more gluttons for the simple punishments he
prescribed.

One of the first offers he received was to enter the service of
the pope, Paul III, as astrologer and physician. He supposed
from this offer that His Holiness had at last come to reading the
two manuscripts, the *Emendation of the Celestial Movements*
and the *Life of Christ* in horoscope form which Archinto had
encouraged him to present nearly ten years before, and perhaps
his other works as well, for it was a matter of form for an
author to present copies of his books to pope, emperor, and
prince. In fact far more subtle machinations were being set in
motion by Tartaglia, who, by declaring his Imperialist sympa-

thies, had wormed his way into the confidence and affection of
Gonzaga, the Governor of Milan. Gonzaga, an ambitious scion
of the Emperor's complex despotism, was by both nature and
training an opponent of Paul. The pontiff's efforts, prolonged
over a dozen years, to secure a lasting peace between France
and Spain and to subjugate the Turks and Reformers, were
looked upon by the Emperor as the dangerous interference of a
senile man (Pope Paul was seventy-nine, liberal, worldly, and
courteous); and Gonzaga, a man of unctuous devotion to the
imperialism that had adopted him, naturally emulated his
Emperor. So when Tartaglia went out of his way to carry to
him a tale that Cardano was seeking to force upon the Pope, by
way of the old man's addiction to astrology, some political
intrigue intended to foster a peaceful settlement between France
and Spain, he listened attentively in spite of the fact that he had
recently arbitrated against Tartaglia in the great public dispute.
Nothing could have been more averse to Gonzaga's ideas—or,
rather, his self-interested adherence to the Emperor's ideas—
than any such intrigue. But he saw that to be forewarned is to
be forearmed. If Cardano could be settled in the papal court as
astrological adviser it would be much easier subsequently to
trace the source of any such intrigue and forestall it, thereby
gaining congratulation and perhaps advancement from the
Emperor. He therefore arranged for the offer to be made—
simply enough, for there were many of the Emperor's minions
in Rome. In the event, Cardano refused the offer. He too saw
the Pope as "A decrepit man, a crumbling wall in the shadow
of which there is no shelter"; but his reasons were merely personal in that he was now in no special need of patronage and
could pick and choose those whose service he entered. He therefore replied courteously to the Pope's emissary to the effect that
His Holiness by his study of astrology had surely raised himself
among the greatest of such scientists and had "no need of help
from such as myself, whose works on the subject are doubtless in
His Holiness's hands, and to which at the moment there is
nothing to be added". Tartaglia was thus cheated of his chance
to entangle Cardano in affairs designed to bring him into disrepute and had to invent some other way.

It was not difficult. Aided by Gonzaga, he arranged a feast in honour of the Pope's emissary before that worthy returned to Rome. A cock-a-hoop young man well wined and dined and subjected to pleasing flattery is a malleable subject, and it was simple enough to implant in the emissary's mind the idea that Cardano had intended to offend His Holiness by his refusal. It was even simpler to produce to him a copy of the *Life of Christ* and convince him that such a horoscope was blasphemous if not heretical. Wisely, they left matters there, thinking that the time for thought afforded by the journey back to Rome would do the rest. Which indeed it did.

Unaware of all this plotting behind his back, Cardano continued his normal life, refusing—or instructing Ferrari to refuse on his behalf—offer after offer from the nobility of half Europe. An offer to which he gave his personal attention because of its royal issue, was that of King Christian III of Denmark. It was a mark of fame indeed that the monarch of so remote a country should make overtures to an Italian physician; but Cardano was not to be tempted. Privately he recorded that he thought the Danes little more than barbarians, and their cold damp climate "no less than an entrance to death's caverns for those of sickly constitution such as myself".[5] (Throughout his life, though his morbid hypochondria diminished, he could never bear to admit himself in good health.) Also, he contemptuously dismissed the Danes as being devoid of culture and therefore having no world of letters in which a man of intellect could pleasurably move, and as being atheists to a man. He was, however, discreet enough not to mention these opinions to the King. He replied that the only reason for his refusal was that he was a widower with children whose education he must supervise and that his plain moral duty was to remain with them and not to travel to a distant country where command over their activities would be impossible.

King Christian's offer carried with it an annual stipend of eight hundred crowns, free maintenance for a household of six people and three horses, and a reminder that all the fees that would accrue from Cardano's medical attentions to the nobles of the court, who naturally would seek his counsel, would probably amount to another eight hundred crowns. It was typical of Cardano that he was not attracted by money; and in any case his salary at Pavia had been raised to four hundred crowns and was being paid regularly, the university having overcome its economic difficulties. But what he found far more attractive than any appointment to pope or king was a request made in a long letter from a fellow physician in an equally remote but far more civilized country, Scotland. It came, by happy chance, at the very moment when it was most welcome. Cardano had for several years been making an intensive study of the treatise on asthma written by the 12th-century physician Moses Maimonides and had supplemented it with a treatise of his own in which he analysed Maimonides' theories and treatment and commented upon them. But it had been, he wrote, a great exasperation to him that no suitable patient had come his way and that he had therefore been unable to test his own theories. Now, the very opportunity he had longed for was put before him.

In writing years later about what turned out to be the triumphant crowning of his medical career, Cardano refers wryly to the request in which it originated as "something more than a letter". With justification. He quotes it in full in *De Vita* and it runs to twenty pages of small print. However, a letter it was in form if not in size, and its content, freed from the prolixities of the salutation and other irrelevant matters was a plea for help. The writer's name was John Cassanate and he was the son of a Spaniard who had settled in Burgundy. (He included a far from brief personal history among the irrelevancies of the letter.) He was now personal physician to John Hamilton, Archbishop of St. Andrews, upon whose illness he sought Cardano's advice. The Archbishop, he said, was a sufferer from chronic asthma. He lengthily described the symptoms and concluded, "I have neither expected at any time his complete cure, nor do I think that the most effectual help will ever bring it about, partly because of the moistness of the air and the strength of the winds, partly also because of his distractions with incessant labours in state affairs, which hang wholly upon him, as it were upon a thread; he is so worried night and day, that in the midst of his vast responsibilities he can hardly rest, still less pay that attention to the care of health which our good Hippocrates highly desired at the hands of sick men and others, as well as of physicians. Now, however, leaving the great tumult of his cares and undertakings, he is about to visit Paris, entirely bent upon attending to his health. But since he has frequently been informed by me of your eminent virtue, your singular erudition and most abundant experience as a practising physician, the Archbishop most eagerly desires your help as the most valid protection that he can obtain against his malady; so that he is persuaded that he will be healed by you as if by the hands of a favouring Apollo. He would spare no cost that would attract you to Paris, and indeed the bearer of this letter will at once advance such expenses and arrange such princely escort as you may wish for your journey. Therefore contrive, I beseech you, that Paris may behold you, for need, according to the precept of Hippocrates, begets urgency".

"Reading this letter", Cardano wrote, "I was in a glow of satisfaction, and I sat down at once to reply that I would go to Paris as soon as I could arrange my affairs. For the expenses of the journey I requested two hundred crowns from Cassanate's envoy, and these I received".

The letter from Cassanate was dated 28th September 1551, but the messenger had had a perilous journey across a Europe confused by war and it had taken him two months to reach Milan. The Archbishop was due in Paris in January, and it was now the end of November. Cardano set out on 12th December. He travelled for the most part on horseback, having scorned the "princely escort" offered by Cassanate, since he was, as he says, not a prince but a doctor—and a doctor in a hurry to boot. The carriages of the day were primitive and slow-moving and required constantly changing teams of horses and frequent attention to offset the ravages made upon them by the extremely bad roads. It was far quicker to use a single horse which could cope with byways and tracks and cross waterways without difficulty. And when one was given a *laissez passer*, as Cardano was, and thus treated with deference and priority in every state, it was possible to demand the post horses that were kept at regular intervals along the highways for the use of official messengers, so that one continually had a fresh animal to travel on. The only exception to this simple and direct method of transport was when, after travelling by way of the Simplon Pass, Sion, and Geneva, he reached Lyons and was met on the outskirts of the city by the governor's seneschal, who told him that his fame would not permit of anything but a civic reception. Cardano therefore entered that city in the style of a prince, drawn in a decorated carriage with outriders and postillion. Of his entry into Lyons he was moved to say, "I recalled the day when I was but a child, and ill, and watched with longing as His Majesty [Louis XII] of France came into Milan".[6]

13

1551–1552

John Hamilton, Archbishop of St Andrews, was the bastard brother of the Earl of Arran who became Regent of Scotland after the death of James V in 1542. James's daughter Mary, who became queen of Scotland and France, was only a week old when he died, and at that time John Hamilton was Abbot of Paisley. He became archbishop after the death of Henry VIII in 1547, by which time Mary had been taken to France to evade Henry's efforts to kidnap her and secure her as the future wife of his son Edward VI. The Archbishop was a zealous partisan of the interests of France and equally staunch in his defence of the church of Rome against the reforms that later were to be established by John Knox. He was a man of strong will and energy and exerted great influence over his brother Lord Arran, whose rule as regent was weak and under continual attack by James V's widow, Mary of Guise, who herself aspired to the regency. It was in fact only by the continual advice and support of the Archbishop that Arran had so far resisted Mary's efforts to throw him from power. But by 1551 the Archbishop's health was failing as a consequence of his unremitting attention to political and ecclesiastical affairs, and his hectic private life. Attacks of asthma occurred with increasing frequency and each time lasted longer. By the time Cassanate wrote in desperation to Cardano they were recurring weekly and lasting twenty-four hours. It was clear that the onslaught of the illness would soon bring him to the point of death. So far it had reduced him to the stage at which he was no longer able to be the power at his brother's elbow, and Mary of Guise, cunningly making the most of the opening thus offered, had forced Arran weakly to commit himself to resign his regency in her favour before the year's end.

All the Archbishop's political designs now rested upon his ability to recover his health sufficiently to prevent Arran from fulfilling his promise. And since he had already been attended without improvement by the physicians of the Emperor Charles and the King of France, who by the protocol of the day had to be invited first, Cardano was the last resort of the sick man who was the power behind the throne of Scotland.

When Cardano arrived in Lyons he found awaiting him a second messenger, who, clearly, had been despatched almost on the heels of the first. He was now asked to await the arrival of Cassanate himself, who would accompany him on the rest of the journey to Paris—"If, indeed, that journey should be necessary, for it may be possible for His Grace the Archbishop to come to Lyons and thereby save your eminent self further tedious travels". This would have suited Cardano very well, for the thought of having to travel further made no appeal to him. But it was not to be. He remained in Lyons for six weeks, hearing no further news. During all that time he was treated with the utmost ceremony and was kept extremely busy by the patients who flocked to him with open purses. He also received an offer from the Frenchman Marshal Brissac—he who had reinforced Archinto's sponsorship of Cardano at the papal court of Paul III—to enter his service as mathematician and designer of war machinery at a thousand crowns a year. But he refused that offer as he had so many others.

At last Cassanate arrived—a small, delicately made, bright-eyed man with a neat beard and a ceaseless flow of conversation matching the prolixity of his letters. He was undone, he said, by the rigours of the journey and handed Cardano a sealed purse of money and a letter from the Archbishop, chattering away while Cardano testily tried to gain information from him on other than the trivial matters of small talk. But Cassanate was not to be drawn; indeed it gradually became clear to Cardano that the chatter was the nervous reaction of a man attempting to postpone an unpleasant task, and he set the purse on the table and looked for enlightenment in the letter. The Archbishop therein explained that he had been "hindered by most serious and urgent and inevitable business and compelled to desist from my intention to leave Edinburgh". (He had in fact

been holding, with the failing strength at his command, the
frail threads of the cat's-cradle on which his brother was still
supported in his regency, realizing that at the present stage of
Mary of Guise's plotting his absence for even a day might
imperil the Hamilton fortunes; so he had struggled even against
the racking attacks of asthma to aid his brother.) The letter
continued along many flowery paths of flattery and begged
Cardano to continue his journey not only to Paris but from
there on to Scotland, using for expenses the three hundred gold
crowns in the purse, with the assurance that for every day he
attended upon the Archbishop he would receive a further
twenty golden growns as a retainer and "any sum that should
be specified, not excluding all the riches of my revenues" if he
effected a cure.[1] Cardano believed—and it may have been partly
true—that the Archbishop had enticed him to France meaning all along that he should go to Edinburgh, but had been
subtle enough to conceal that intention in the letter sent to
Milan, where Cardano might well have had second thoughts
about making the journey at all. In fact, though travelling in
general and Scotland in particular were distasteful to Cardano,
he would, he says, have accepted the commission anyway
because of the medical interest of the case.[2] Much to the relief
of the dithering Cassanate he therefore agreed to go on to Scotland with as much speed as possible, adding acidly, "There was
a great urgency about His Grace's illness which has now melted
away in delays : if Death, who can be as fleet as he wills, is
not to be awaiting us on the threshold, let us travel while we
parley".

Which they did. It was by now spring and they took to the
river for their highway. The Loire valley was probably at its
best; but Cardano had no eye for scenery. The two doctors
spent all their time "parleying" about the Archbishop's asthma.
Cardano was most anxious to know many things about the case
outside the list of symptoms he had been given in Cassanate's
letter. The Archbishop's hours of sleep, his diet, his exercise, his
sexual habits, the condition of his living-quarters, his clothing,
whether he sat or stood for most of his working hours, the temperature and humidity of the Edinburgh air—all these matters
and a dozen others were carefully enquired into by Cardano.

And it is easy to see why. Maimonides, the Jewish physician who had prepared his treatise on asthma in 1190 after being called to a high-born patient in Alexandria, had divided his observations into chapters dealing with general conduct for the asthmatic, diet, preparation of food, and drinks that may be taken, the respiration and emotional processes, evacuation in its various forms, sleeping, bathing and coitus, and the various drugs and remedies with notes on their preparation. His approach had been simple and direct. But in the centuries intervening between his time and Cardano's the so-called magic of sorcerers and alchemists had obscured in clouds of hocus-pocus much of the basic simplicity of medical practice. Cardano's theory of the treatment of asthma was an extension of Maimonides'. He believed that afflictions of a bronchitic, asthmatic, or phthisic nature were organically incurable but could be relieved by a proper regimen; and it was in anticipation of imposing such a regimen upon the Archbishop that he made such detailed enquiries of Cassanate. They produced replies that did not surprise him. The Archbishop was not only an intelligent and energetic worker in all his political and ecclesiastical causes : he enjoyed to excess the high living that his large income provided. Huge meals, gallons of wine, irregular hours, and liaisons with women that in every sense of the phrase became him ill, had wrought havoc with his body. It had apparently not occurred to Cassanate that less excess in every direction might be beneficial. But that does not mean that he was stupid. It was an age of fleshpots; virility had to be forced if it was not naturally in evidence; and it was the general attitude of physicians that the body was meant to endure anything and everything. Cardano was exceptional in reverting to the teaching of earlier men who had a higher concern for human machinery.

The delay occasioned by waiting for Cassanate could not be made up. It was in fact elongated by the civic ceremonies that awaited Cardano in Paris. Aimar de Ranconet, a lawyer in the Fourth Chamber of Accounts in the Paris parliament, had made arrangements for a banquet and a sightseeing tour; Nicolas Legrand, the royal physician who had already been consulted by Cassanate, had arranged several conferences of doctors. It was impossible to escape. His hosts would allow no such thing.

Fretful though he was at the delay, Cardano enjoyed his stay in Paris, though he found the streets "always full of dirt, emitting stench, and the air unwholesome, the population being at the same time dense". Of the sightseeing, he says that Legrand, "Being physician also to the monks of St Dionysius, took us to their noble church, distant about three miles from Paris, and famed throughout the whole world. There, when we had seen the sepulchres of kings, statues, and other marble ornaments, I studied carefully the horn of an unicorn. I handled it and measured it, and among all the king's treasures there was nothing that appeared to be so precious as that rare and perfect horn". As before, when he had the encounter with the wizard who supposedly drove from him the evil spirit and had to be rewarded with powdered horn, it seems that the scientific side of his mind is at variance with superstition. Several times in *De Varietate Rerum* he mentions the alleged curative effects of alicorn; but nowhere does he ever say he prescribes it for a patient.

Of his journey in general he remarks that throughout he never once had to show his *laissez passer* : his name was enough. "Serious war was at that time raging between the Emperor Charles and the King of France. All things were being destroyed with fire and sword; infants and women were being slain. Yet although it was known that I was a subject of the enemy Emperor; yet so far was I from suffering any harm, that I was received in the best spirit by the nobles. So much was thought due to learning and good name by the French nobility. The enemy protects an alien lest he perish miserably in the hands of his own people".[3] For such protection the governor of the coast provinces, when Cardano and Cassanate came to Boulogne, had them attended by an escort of fourteen horse and twenty foot soldiers to Calais. There they went aboard a French galley. This was Cardano's first experience of travel by sea and he did not relish it. The stench was more than could be blown away by the Channel breezes, and he soon discovered that it rose from below decks where the galley slaves were compelled to urinate and defacate as they sat chained to the benches. "The benches are four feet wide covered with sacking stuffed with wool over which are thrown sheepskins which reach to the deck be-

neath them. The officer who is master of the galley slaves remains aft with the captain to receive his orders. There are two
under officers, one amidships and one at the prow; and all of
them are armed with whips, with which they flog the totally
naked bodies of the slaves. When the captain gives the order to
row, the officer gives the signal with a silver whistle which hangs
on a cord round his neck. The signal is repeated by the under
officers and very soon all the fifty oars strike the water as if one.
Imagine six men chained to a bench as naked as they were
born, one foot on the stretcher, the other raised and placed on
the bench in front of them, holding in their hands an oar of
immense weight, stretching their bodies towards the after part of
the galley with arms extended to push the loom of the oar clear
of the backs of those in front of them, who are in the same
attitude. They plunge the blades of the oars into the water and
throw themselves back, falling onto the seat which bends beneath their weight. Sometimes the galley slaves row thus ten,
twelve, even twenty hours at a stretch, without the slightest
respite or rest. On these occasions the officers will go round,
putting into the mouths of the wretched rowers pieces of bread
soaked in wine to prevent them from fainting."[4]

The delays that had made Cardano so impatient but to
which he had become resigned, had taken the time forward into
the summer of 1552. The galley sailed round the southeast coast
and dropped anchor in the Thames on 3rd June, and the journey to Edinburgh took another three weeks. So it was not until
29th June that the Archbishop at last met Cardano.

His clinical notes on the case occupy forty pages of close print in
double columns. He describes his patient as of middle size, with
a thin neck, a deep chest, and a coarse red skin that sweated
freely. There is a great deal of unsalubrious detail regarding the
expectorated sputum, and many conclusions based on the
assumption that "vapours" and fluids rise from the lungs to the
brain, drawn there by the rarified atomsphere of that organ.
Once there, the "vapours" are exhaled through the skin, but the
fluids remain. They turn thick and corrupt and in time by their
increasing weight descend through the windpipe to the lungs
again, where their viscosity and bulk cause the irritation that

makes the patient cough painfully in the effort to expel them.[5]
These conclusions today appear quaint, risible. They are based
on guesswork, they prove ignorance of the body's mechanism.
They assume two definite conditions of the brain—"hot" and
"cold"—over which there was great argument in Paris at the
conferences Cardano attended, he maintaining that the Archbishop's was of the "hot" order while the others argued for
"cold". However nonsensical such an assumption appears, there
is no doubt that Cardano's determination to treat for a "hot"
brain was, partly by happy chance and partly by the gropings
of a mind intuitively turned in the right direction, of a kind that
undoubtedly would relieve the asthmatic conditions. The other
doctors' assumption of the disease being seated in a "cold" brain
had resulted in the Archbishop being confined to smoky, stifling
rooms that did nothing but irritate his bronchial tubes, with a
brazier of burning peat or charcoal even in the carriage in
which he was transported from one place to another. He was
masked against any fresh air and was allowed only scalding
foods and mulled wines so that his temperature should be kept
high enough to make him sweat copiously and continuously. It
is not surprising that treatment of this kind, combined with high
living, had brought him to a state at which he was scarcely
living at all.

Cardano immediately switched the regimen to one that in
basis was completely opposite. The root cause of the disease
being the unhealthily high temperature of the brain, he said, the
head and body should be purged. To do this he prescribed, *inter
alia*: an inhalant of elaterium in goat's milk; application to the
skull of an ointment of ship's tar, mustard, euphorbium, honey
of Anathardus and blister-fly; the washing of the head in warm
water to which ashes had been added, followed by a cold
shower and mild massage with cool dry cloths; and a compound
of peaches and sugar of violets washed down with the milk of a
well nourished ass that had been fed on corn and barley supplemented with rose blossoms, mallow, and beet. ("And it is of the
gravest importance," he added, "that the ass should have foaled
recently and should run daily with her foal in the meadows".)
The order of the Archbishop's day now was to be completely
different and strictly observed. "His Grace, having performed

his first morning duties, should next comb his head with an ivory comb to comfort the brain, anoint his spine and chest with oil of sweet almonds, and walk for a short time in some pleasant spot, not sunny. At nine he should break fast with the liver of a fowl seasoned with two grains of ginger, followed by bread soaked in gravy, and two ounces of white wine. That being eaten, the stewed flesh of the chicken and wine from four or five more times up to ten ounces. Then to rest and amuse himself (but not with harlots) until noon. For four hours then His Grace may attend to business but should not write any letters with his own hand and should as much as possible avoid trouble. At four he should ride for an hour upon a gentle horse and having returned should recline upon his bed while he gives an audience to those who desire speech with him. By no means should he be outdoors at twilight. At seven he should sup on a spoonful of pure honey with bread, broth, and ass's milk; and at eight he should go to bed and secure ten hours of continuous sleep. The nature of His Grace's bed, and the manner of his lying upon it are of the greatest importance. No circumstances should allow a feather mattress to be used, for it heats the spine and causes matter straightaway to ascend to the brain. The mattress and pillow should be of silk stuffed with finely chopped dry straw or dried seaweed, and he should never lie upon his back but on his face or side, with a hand to his stomach. By this means he will find relief from a discharge through the mouth, while the hand upon the stomach will aid digestion."

There was a great deal more, and it was all written painstakingly by hand for the Archbishop's reference in a document separate from the clinical notes intended for publication, the *Consilia Medica*. Every eventuality seemingly was taken into consideration so that Cardano's actual presence should not be necessary once he had established the success of the treatment. This he did within forty days. He personally attended the preparation of the Archbishop's meals, was on hand to see him rise and take his exercise, and could give him relief with inhalants and perfumes when the coughing bouts occurred. Also he could soothe his choleric temper, which was much in evidence during the early days of the treatment on account of his reluctance to quit the fleshpots that to him seemed a necessity. Cardano,

however, held the whip hand; for to bring his patient to heel he
had only to say—and indeed many times said—that he would
as soon go as stay. For Hamilton found the treatment beneficial
from the very beginning; and after a fortnight or so could
scarcely bear to let Cardano from his sight. By that time the
incidence of the bouts had greatly diminished thereby giving his
body something of a chance to recover of its natural resources—
a recovery that Cardano assisted with nourishing foods such as
turtle or tortoise soup, distilled liquor or snails, and barley
water. Cardano being himself of no easy temper, it is pleasing to
imagine the two gentlemen exasperated with each other but
bound to pacify each other with smooth words—the patient in
case he should lose his physician, the physician in case he should
raise his patient's choler to an injurious extent. It was perhaps
in this spirit that Cardano cast for the Archbishop a horoscope—for which, considering his fame as an astrologer, Hamilton not surprisingly asked him—that was encouraging. In fact,
Cardano saw nothing but gloom in the Archbishop's stars. And
he was to be proved tragically right. But he drew a chart which
revealed mild perils in 1554 and later dangers of enmity to be
avoided, but otherwise was most optimistic of the future. There
was considerable psychological understanding at work here.
Optimism is always a splendid asset for a sick man; and the
truth could hardly have left him optimistic. Cardano therefore
allowed his astrologer's conscience to tussle with his physician's
conscience and that latter one to win.

It was just as well that he did. Encouraged by the very stars
themselves to be confident in his own recovery, the Archbishop
made splendid progress. Cardano stayed on for some while yet,
drawing to the suite that had been provided for him in the
Archbishop's palace a great number of noble patients who
sought his advice. In advising and treating them he made a
great deal of money—"In a single day, nineteen golden
crowns". But his greatest satisfaction came with the visit of an
envoy of the king, young Edward VI, who had recently recovered from measles and smallpox and had developed an infection of the lungs that had baffled his doctors. "It has come to
Our ears," the envoy read from the King's letter, "that you, the
great and beloved physician Gerolamo Cardano, have raised

from a death bed our holy Archbishop of Scotland and have a
great skill in treating these ills of the chest. Therefore at your
pleasure wait upon us when you return to London."[7] King or no
king however, Cardano would not leap without proper consideration from the bedside of one patient to that of another. He stayed
in the end seventy-five days in Scotland and was rewarded most
lavishly by the Archbishop and all the noblemen whom he had
attended. In addition to the agreed stipend of twenty crowns a
day he received a *pour boire* of eighteen hundred crowns and a
gold chain worth a hundred and twenty-five crowns; also an
"ambling good-tempered horse for the comfort of my journey to
London". He said goodbye to the Archbishop and Cassanate on
12th September, and he and his servants were escorted by a
troop of cavalry the entire way to London so that Cardano's
treasury of boxes containing some five thousand crowns in gold
should not be stolen.

At the court in London Cardano was welcomed and sheltered
by Sir John Cheke, tutor and chamberlain of the exchequer to
the young king. He very quickly learnt that the letter summon-
ing him as a physician had in truth been meant to inveigle him
into providing an astrological prediction of the king's future for
the benefit of the unscrupulous Duke of Northumberland, John
Dudley, who had been appointed Protector. Such a forecast
would of course have aided Dudley in his unprincipled ambitions, and it says much for Cardano's fame as an astrologer that
he should have been called upon to play his part in English
political manoeuvring at that crucial period of history. He did
not, however, see himself as a pawn in that complex game. He
agreed to provide the required horoscope but secretly determined that whatever truth the stars might reveal he would
adjust that truth so that he would not himself become involved
in court intrigues. It was as well that he did. "The stars made of
the king's life that it had but a few more months to run, though
he was not yet sixteen years of age". The stars were only too
correct. Edward VI, always sickly in body, died less than a year
later. Had Cardano revealed that prophecy, the conniving Dudley might well have been aided in his plot to put the puppet
queen, Lady Jane Grey, upon the throne. Instead, he shrewdly
provided a far less dangerous forecast. "Speaking generally of

the King's life, its whole duration will be of fifty-six years and beyond to an extent not clearly revealed. He will be found to be steadfast, firm, chaste, intelligent, patient in trouble, mindful of both injuries and benefits, one demanding reverence and seeking his own. He will prove wise beyond measure and thereby win the admiration of the world; prudent and highminded; fortunate and indeed a second Solomon".

Having entered briefly upon the English scene and by a tiny measure changed the course of history—ironically by falsifying the course of the stars—Cardano now set out for home.

14

1552

A hitherto scarcely visible facet of Cardano's nature now reveals itself As I have said,* the autobiographical passages in *De Libris Propriis* relating to his student days are concerned mainly to catalogue his physical features and deficiencies. One infers from the sparse details he gives of his sexual proclivities that he experienced cunnilingus and fellatio, both heterosexually and homosexually, before he experienced normal coitus. But it is by no means certain. There are occasional references to his voyeurism and self-abuse and some harping on his impotence—which, as we know, was cured by the dream in which Lucia first appeared to him. But clearly he thinks these matters of small interest. (The 16th century was as salacious as our own, but there was far less selfconsciousness about it.) It is therefore mildly surprising to see unfolded the story—or, rather, the edges of the story; for he is never explicit about it—of his association with an English boy, William.

He had, it is clear, a high regard for the English as a race—body and character alike. "[They are] much as we [Italians] are in figure, but not so ruddy; they are broadchested, many are tall, they are quick in anger and dreadful in war. Greedy in food and drink (but not so much as the Germans), and with great intellects among them. In nature they are faithful, liberal, brave, and ambitious; and the Scots are of the English [sic] the most courageous of all and will take a piper with them as they go to the stake, who plays them, dancing, to their death".[1] This high regard he wished to implement by taking back with him to Milan an English boy. And at Dover, while he was awaiting a wind for his ship, he fell in with a family who lodged him and

*p. 29.

who had a boy of twelve years whom they were anxious, they said, "to launch upon the world". There was evidently some handing over of cash, whereupon William was his. The very next morning, the wind standing fair, the ship set sail and was away, with Cardano and the boy, plus servants and treasury, safely aboard. Only then did Cardano discover that William spoke only English and that it was therefore impossible to communicate with him. This seems to have soured him and turned him against the boy. "I began to try to make him repent of his agreement to come with me by disgusting him of me by whipping him on the bare skin. But this he enjoyed, and I too, so that it came to be turn and turn about".[2] This sado-masochistic vignette is all Cardano reveals of the relationship for a long time; and he never indeed reveals anything overtly at all. But there is a wealth of passionate emotion to be inferred from the silence between the first and last chapters of the story, as we shall see. Meanwhile, we continue with him on his journey home.

He was, as he had told the Archbishop, longing to return to his beloved children. And to that end he had refused Hamilton's pressing invitation to stay on as a guest in Scotland. The shortest way back to Milan was of course through France, and that had been Cardano's intended route. He had indeed promised to attend upon many rich but sickly noblemen when he passed through Paris again. But while staying with Sir John Cheke in London he had heard that France was overrun with bandits bred out of the conditions of war, and that these would give short shrift to any man attended richly by servants and carrying with him so much treasure. He therefore decided sensibly that the longest way round might well be the shortest way home in terms of safety, and planned to go through the Netherlands to Cologne and into Italy by way of Basel and Zurich.

In Basel occurred a sinister incident the meaning of which was to remain a mystery for some time. At Mulhouse he had sent ahead of him a courier to choose and arrange lodging with some learned person in Basel. The courier awaited him on the outskirts of the town and told him with an immense degree of flattery that the most distinguished man in Basel, Gemma Fracantiano, awaited him with all ceremony. "In what field is the

excellent lord distinguished?" Cardano enquired. "In the very
field in which your honour will soon gain notoriety", the courier
said with much sycophantic washing of the hands. He then gave
Cardano careful directions, warned him that every other house
in Basel was a hovel unsuitable for a gentleman of his status,
and unctuously retreated backward out of Cardano's presence as
if from the throne of a king. Cardano may have been mildly
surprised at the insistence with which he was enjoined to lodge
at that house and no other; but he made no protest. On his way
there, however, he chanced to meet a scholarly friend from
Milan, Guglielmo Gratalaro, who had been living in Basel for
some years. He was horrified to learn that Cardano intended to
lodge with Fracantiano—who, he said, was no learned man but
a spy for the Inquisition whose real name was Peter Titelmann.
Gratalaro's manner was so secretive and his concern so great
that Cardano accepted his warning not to tarry for a moment
longer in Basel—a decision that was probably reinforced by the
further news imparted to him by Gratalaro that a case of plague
had been notified in the town. He is sparse with the details of
this incident, perhaps because he thought little of it and was
concerned mainly to humour his old friend.[3] But the circumstances are very like those prevailing in Germany when the
Gestapo reigned. And indeed Titelmann was to become one of
the most notorious persecutors of the Reformation. In the
Netherlands his infamous deeds terrified rich and poor alike,
and his pursuit of those he chose to suspect of even the mildest
forms of heresy was unrelenting. No doubt in this early part of
his career, in 1552, he was learning the technique of eaves-
dropping and the subtleties of inducing his victims to say in all
innocence words he would later twist to guilt. Cardano was
fortunate to quit Basel without crossing his path. But he did not
entirely elude his intricate web of operations; and the signifi-
cance of the incident, and its instigator, would later be revealed.

Cardano returned to Milan along the Gallarate road on 3 January 1553. He had been away a year and three weeks. Crowds
turned out to welcome him—not the official crowds that made
obeisances to prince or governor, but the cheery crowds who remembered him as a worthy kinsman. Again he makes a contrast

between past and present—though not a bitter one. "How different this arrival from the former one when I was with a young and trusting wife and we came from Gallarate as paupers! Now they put up bowers for me to pass under and my treasure-boxes are great enough to be drawn on a cart flanked by guardsmen. Where I was despised I am now the chief physician, where I was unknown my skills in medicine, numbers, the stars, wisdom, and machines are everywhere discussed. Honours and awards have been flung at me till I grow weary of them. Sovereigns of church, palace and battlefield have summoned me to their aid. This is what the stars foretold. It is not of my doing".

On the contrary, it was very much of his doing. Whatever the stars may foretell, they do not wield the instruments of achievement.

15

1552–1556

During his absence the legal disputes over Fazio's inheritance had been resolved. It had turned out that there was property and money that no one had known about till the lawyers had begun their delvings and arguments. Since Fazio was not of the disposition to make secret caches, one can only assume that he had from time to time made investments and loans he had subsequently forgotten about. Cardano is not enlightening on the subject; but he notes with irony the fact that "at a time of fortune more fortune is added". And he observes too that his own home life at the time he was growing up would have been happier if Fazio had remembered that he had money to lay hands on and where it was. "Our rent-masters were forever in pursuit and I was forever bewildered as to where I would spend my day and open my eyes on the morrow".

His own children had had little of such insecurity and might therefore have been expected to flourish in every way. And indeed Cardano beheld them and reunited himself to them with admiration and love on his return to Milan. Perhaps he was screened from suspicions of their true nature by doting affection; perhaps he understood more than he admitted. Writing in old age, when all the troubles were over, he is reticent, as if seeing some blame in himself. If there was any, it is difficult to place it.

Giovanni was now nineteen years old, slightly lame because of his subjoined toes, slightly crook-backed, and with more of a sinister manner than Cardano sees or cares to admit. To him the boy is all things a firstborn son should be. "Except in bodily shape, where he lacks the grace of perfection, he is of the greatest accomplishment".[2] That was written on the night of the arrival back in Milan. It is a scrap of journal that has survived. Twenty years later Cardano's feeling was very different. "He never even had the wit to deceive me", he says of the boy. Mistakenly. Giovanni had wit for little else but deception. He was at the time of Cardano's return revealing remarkable obtuseness in passing even the preliminary examinations that should lead to his baccalaureat. Contrasted with the brilliant mind of Ferrari, who had been coaching him, his was dross. But he managed to deceive Cardano—and the deception must have been supported by Ferrari—into believing that he had suffered only from obstructive examiners. Remembering the difficulties of his own passage through the university, Cardano gave Giovanni the benefit of the doubt. The youth was in any case a fawning proponent of his own affairs. He had a smooth charm that simultaneously attracted but at the same time seemed to scorn sympathy for his lameness and deformity, leaving the sympathizer the more certain of his patient suffering in the face of misfortune. No doubt it was easy to draw upon his father's compassion. Had not the boy been the subject of waspish intervention on the very day of his baptism? "I had daily apprehensions about him, but I put them aside in my joy in seeing him again, strengthening my belief that if only a failure to gain his baccalaureat was to be accounted for, then there was little indeed to fear".[4] There, Cardano was again writing in old age. One can almost hear him sigh as he reviews his indulgences to a son who was to prove worthless, indeed worse than worthless

As for Chiara, she was now seventeen. Thaddaea reported well of her; and it appears that she kept her eyes cast down, blushed easily, and had a respectful manner. Thaddaea, however, as we know, was often away from Cardano's house in Milan (which had been rebuilt during his absence) looking after her own household in Sacco. Formidable and sharp-eyed though she was, Chiara found no difficulty in bribing and blackmailing the servants to give suitable accounts of her movements during Thaddaea's absences. In this she was aided by Giovanni. The social evenings and chaperoned walks proper for a maid of Chiara's age and station were all recorded in the day-books so carefully inspected by the children's grandmother. And certainly the records did not lie : they merely omitted. The elder Chiara's characteristics were repeating themselves in her daughter. But commercial licentiousness had become magnified into something approaching nymphomania. Before she was sixteen the girl had seduced her brother. Giovanni, nothing loath, had lain with her and she had become pregnant. Just as his mother attempted to abort Gerolamo, so his daughter attempted to abort the child of this incestuous union, and was successful—though at the cost of her fertility. But of that she was scornful. She had no wish for children : only for the instrument of their conception. Her lusts, even at that age when her father took his greatest delight in her and proudly displayed her at the musical entertainments he had resumed immediately on his return, were enormous. In that she was typical of the epoch. But she made of them something nastily furtive, disguised by simpering innocence. "There was nought of honesty at all in her whoring", said a contemporary.[5] So again Cardano was deceived and is reticent about the actual time when he came to realize his daughter's true character. It may well be that he could not bear to write about the wound the realization made in his heart.

The little boy, Aldo, was only ten years old. He was the child to whom the stars had been so liberal in promises of genius, fame, wealth, the confidence of princes. "Genius he had", Cardano writes of him bitterly; "but not of the order of a father's desire". The exact nature of that genius was at that time developing in the boy; and if Cardano saw the onset of corruption in Aldo's brutal treatment of the household animals, he probably attributed it to the mischievous impulses of a child.

Such, then, were the characters of Cardano's children. And their acts were shortly to display proof that could not pass unnoticed by even the most blindly devoted of fathers.

There was also in the household now the English boy William. Unable to speak the language he was none the less easily conducted along the paths of evil by the three Cardano children, since corruption has a language of its own. A fascinating tale could doubtless be made of the conniving and intrigue into which he was drawn. There are available the materials with which might be erected a first-class fiction. But the known details are few. One infers—not from Cardano but from other contemporary sources—that the boy was immediately seduced by Chiara; that he was taught to lie and steal as easily as he picked up a rudimentary knowledge of Italian; that he became the henchman of Giovanni in that young man's evil designs. But until the climatic events that brought disgrace and punishment in their wake one cannot follow very closely the daily machinations of the offspring who were supposed to bring Cardano the rewards of paternity. But it is safe to say that as his love for his children gradually foundered on the crags of their wickedness, so his affection for William increased. It was evidently an affection basically sexual, for he mentions incidentally "the pleasures of beating"; but he also reproaches himself for neglecting his duty to the boy. "He was so loved by me that he could not have been loved better; and that made me feel more heavily that I appeared to be deficient in my duty to him. But in the meantime, so many impediments were raised in my way by my children, that I could attend to little else. Now one troubled me, now the other, sometimes both at once".[6]

There were public as well as domestic troubles. No man reaches the pinnacles of fame without someone attempting to belittle him. Another scholar, Julius Caesar Scaliger, famous in those days and later, mounted a great literary attack on one of Cardano's books, *De Subtilitate*. This was a popular scientific work that had already run into six editions, and Scaliger slashed at it with abuse and ridicule, revealing in the process considerable wit and concealing his own envy of Cardano's success. The publication of the attack flung Cardano into the storm centre of a great controversy; but he maintained a dignified silence, believing that the success of *De Subtilitate* needed no defence. His silence, aided by the slowness of wartime communications between Italy and France (where Scaliger lived), built up the conviction in Scaliger's mind that Cardano had died. The conviction may well have been fostered by practical jokers. At all events, it was not a conviction that Scaliger cared for, since it carried the implication that by his cruel attack he had brought about the death by shock of one of the great men of the day. Envious and cowardly though he was, he was no murderer. He set to at once to try to make amends by publishing a panegyric on Cardano's work and fame. In that way, he supposed, he would escape censure. In fact he got precisely the reward he deserved. His eulogy eventually—actually at the end of 1555—reached Milan, where it gave the far-from-dead Cardano a great deal of amusement. He then wrote a refutation of Scaliger's attack, addressed insultingly not to him by name but merely to "a calumniator who committed more errors than he attempted to correct and whose only object in attacking my reputation was to acquire one of his own".[7] Since Scaliger had by now become the ridiculous butt of the pranksters who had built up the esoteric joke of Cardano's death, he was doubly shamed by the refutation. Cardano may well be said to have won that battle having fired only the single shot. But for the two years in which he held his fire his public reputation was heavily assailed in the broadsheets, ballads, quips, and comedies that in those days served the purpose that daily newspapers would later fulfil.

As for domestic troubles, these mounted toward their climax in 1556 with the achievement by Giovanni (certainly with the influential backing of his father) of a doctor's degree. Another step toward the climax was trodden by Chiara in the same year by her marriage to a young Milanese patrician named Bartolomeo Sacco. Cardano convinced himself that he saw in these events the fulfilment of the parental hopes that had long been eluding him. For a man in his position—famous, rich, revered as doctor, mathematician, philosopher, astrologist, and inventor of ingenious machines, it was proper that his children should reflect his status; and he was willing enough to see what he wanted to see. The evidence of his children's worthlessness, to which he had so often blinded himself, could now be concealed beneath new hopes that they were following straighter paths. "I am overjoyed that my daughter is to marry", he wrote; "and she shall have a handsome dowry".[8] He was even more pleased that Giovanni could now practise as a doctor and was a member of the College of Physicians. He thrust to the back of his mind the knowledge that only his own influence had aided Giovanni in getting his degree. He had only scraped through the examination, and in every way that it was possible to cheat he had done so. As for Chiara, the deceptions she had visited upon her father as to her true character had long worn thin. But

Cardano optimistically thought that marriage would settle her into a way of life more becoming.

Alas for his hopes and self-deceptions! Far from applying himself industriously to his practice, Giovanni made nothing of it at all. His wretchedly inadequate attempts at study had in any case been no more than a pretence that he was engaged in worthy work rather than in the evil designs that in fact filled his life. Now that he had achieved the insignia of a doctor he was delighted to put honest work aside and revert to those paths along which his distorted mind directed his twisted body. There he moved with the natural instincts of an evil-doer, planning with associates who were as corrupt as himself the crimes of robbery, blackmail, and procurement that gave them, in beholding the downfall of their victims, the satisfaction of a petty authority similar to that enjoyed today by gangs of hooligans. Amid the flux of religious and political corruption that was the order of the day no opportunities were lacking. The Emperor Charles V had abdicated in 1556, but his son Philip, sometime husband of Mary Tudor, had continued the oligarchic policy that intended the complete destruction of those zealous enough to persist in flaunting the "heresies" of the Reformation. It was possible, indeed simple, to sell one's dearest friend to the agents of the Inquisition on a trumped-up charge of heresy. Noblemen were prepared to advance their own causes over the destroyed characters of their rivals. Within the curia there were always to be found those priests who acquired their riches by the sale of pardons and to whom a continual flow of information was essential. It was a hegemony in which treachery flourished like an orchid in a hothouse. Giovanni and his kind were well served.

It was inevitable that involvement with villains should bring disaster as well as advantage. With Giovanni disaster took the form of marriage—a marriage forced upon him by a family, the Seronis, who were as unscrupulous as he was and never hesitated to turn fortuitous discovery to their own benefit. They had somehow secured proof that Giovanni had administered the poison that had caused the death of a minor official in the city's administration. They cared nothing for the official's death or the machinery of plotting in which he had been a tiny cog; indeed they would have brought his death about themselves if the payment had been adequate. But they saw at once that here was a ready-made tool to lever them into a luxurious and parasitic life. Threatening Giovanni with exposure to the College of Physicians, they offered him the alternative of marriage to Brandonia, one of the four unmarried women of the family. The marriage was to carry with it the dowry of free accommodation and support for the entire Seroni ménage—an aged crone of a mother, three more unmarried daughters, and three hobbledehoy sons who filled in the time between their mischievous activities by selling their services as mercenary soldiers. Giovanni quite lightly accepted the terms in which they proposed to sell him their silence. It seemed to him a comical situation. Brandonia was far from attractive and equally far from being virgin; but he had no objection to marrying her to secure his own safety; the marriage vows could be made as lightly as the Hippocratic oath; and although he of course had no means to provide the essential dowry, he had no compunction whatever in assuring the Seroni family that they would be welcome in his father's house.

In that he was, understandably, mistaken. Cardano's anger was unbounded. On the very morning on which Giovanni announced to him what was intended to be a *fait accompli* he had had "oppressive visitations of the spirits". The whole house had trembled as if with an earthquake and he had seen in the palm of his own right hand "the semblance of a bloody dagger". These occurrences were to him the most awful of warnings. Following close upon them came Giovanni's announcement. It was not to be expected that Cardano would receive the news with equanimity. Nor did he. His mind was flurried, his heart was filled with bitterness. He absolutely refused shelter and food either to Giovanni or his new-found family of parasites. The door was flung to against them and guards were employed to beat them off if they should attempt entry. He thus severed all but the most vestigial connexion between himself and his once-loved firstborn. His act of rejection was the source of a burden of self-reproach which as long as he lived he was never to overcome. But in the anguish of the moment he saw nothing but moral righteousness in his act.

16

1554-1560

Amid all the confusion and chagrin of those years that gave
with one hand and took away with the other, there was great
joy for Cardano in a letter he received from Archbishop Hamilton at the end of 1554.

Your two most welcome letters, written in former months, I
received through the hands of an English merchant; another
was brought by the lord bishop of Dundee, with the Indian
balsam. Your last letter I had from Scoto, with your most
choice commentaries on the very difficult work of Ptolemy.
To all these I have three or four times amply and abundantly
replied. For I had addressed very many letters to you, but
am uncertain whether they have reached your hands.

Now, however, I have given orders to a servant whom
you know,* and who is travelling to Rome, that he shall pay
a visit to your excellency, and, saluting you in my name,
thank you, not only for your various and very welcome little
gifts, but also for my health, that is in great part restored, for
the almost complete subjugation of my disease, for strength
regained; in fine, I may say, for life recovered. All those good
things, and this body of mine itself, I hold as received from
you. From the time when I had your medicines, prescribed
and prepared with so much art and dexterity, and have
followed your régime of living, the disease that is peculiar to
me has made its visits with much less frequency and violence;
the accustomed attacks now scarcely occur once a month, or
once in two months; then too they are not urgent and pressing, as they used to be, but are felt very slightly.

* He was the Archbishop's chamberlain.

It would look like ingratitude (and I confess to it) if I did not acknowledge all those many and great benefits and send you back thanks. But now I despatch to you a living letter (namely, this Michael), and entreat and pray your excellency, from my heart, that if I can be of use to you in anything, with aid, service, or money, you will send word to me by him; he will, without delay, send me intelligence, and the moment I have tidings of it, consider the thing done.

Besides, Master John Cassanate, the physician, went home last year to his father's house, and has not yet returned. A man certainly worthy of great name and honour, whose daily offices and house companionship are very pleasant to me. I would much urge and beg your excellency not to fall short of your usual kindness in writing to me, that the separation of our bodies may not be a separation of our minds, but that we may be always present to each other. I wish you, in my name, to salute those who are of your household. Farewell. From our metropolitan seat of Saint Andrew. October 1554.

Truly the letter was a joy and an encomium to his virtue as a physician. Among other things to be credited to those years his work, in which he never slackened, was a permanent if exhausting pleasure. His meetings and correspondences with scholars were an extension of that pleasure. The boy William was increasingly the object of his love. But when added up and compared with the sum of the wretched troubles brought to him by Tartaglia and the reprobate children in whom he had hoped in his later years to find comfort, the total showed a decided favour on the side of misfortune.

During the years in which Cardano's fame remained at its glowing apogee, Tartaglia worked his designs with subtle malevolence. He waited to strike, and no doubt saw many opportunities to do so. The great controversy inaugurated by Scaliger's attack would certainly have provided one. But with the instinctive timing of the natural schemer he withheld his hand. It was as if he sensed that there would be a better, more potent, moment. And even out of his own malevolence he could not have contrived a more effective delay.

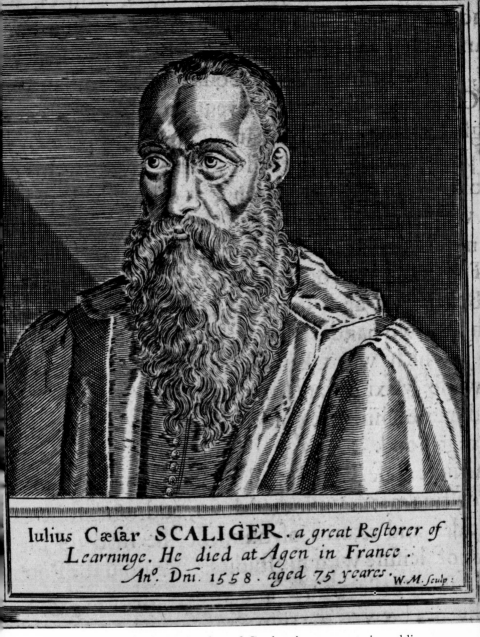

Iulius Cæſar **SCALIGER**. *a great Reſtorer of
Learninge. He died at Agen in France.
Anᵒ. Dñi. 1558. aged 75 yeares.* W.M. Sculp:

Julius Caesar Scaliger, another of Cardano's opponents in public
mathematical debate

HIERONYMI CAR

DANI, PRÆSTANTISSIMI MATHE-

MATICI, PHILOSOPHI, AC MEDICI,

ARTIS MAGNÆ,

SIVE DE REGVLIS ALGEBRAICIS,

Lib.unus. Qui & totius operis de Arithmetica, quod

OPVS PERFECTVM

inscripsit,est in ordine Decimus.

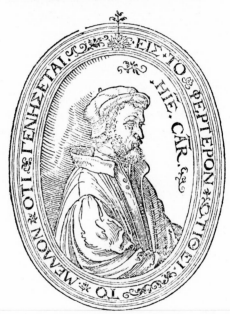

HAbes in hoc libro,studiose Lector,Regulas Algebraicas (Itali, de la Cos
sa uocant) nouis adinuentionibus,ac demonstrationibus ab Authore ita
locupletatas,ut pro pauculis antea uulgò tritis,iam septuaginta euaserint. Ne=
q̃ solum , ubi unus numerus alteri,aut duo uni,uerum etiam,ubi duo duobus,
aut tres uni equales fuerint,nodum explicant.   Hunc aũt librum ideo seor=
sim edere placuit,ut hoc abstrusissimo, & planè inexhausto totius Arithmeti
cæ thesauro in lucem eruto , & quasi in theatro quodam omnibus ad spectan
dum exposito, Lectores incitarétur,ut reliquos Operis Perfecti libros, qui per
Tomos edentur,tanto auidius amplectantur,ac minore fastidio perdiscant.

The title page of Cardano's *Ars Magna*, 1545

Immediately upon returning from Britain, Cardano had resumed his professorship at Pavia. Any appointment he wished could have been his for the asking, there or at Milan. Probably, ineed, in any city in Italy. Offers of Rectorships and Chairs abounded. But the Chair of Medicine at Pavia gave him exactly what he needed : a position in which he could encourage others in the profession in which he himself had excelled in wisdom; the pleasure of making his *alma mater* the centre of the medical world; and time to continue his practice and the writing of his books. Money flowed into his coffers from copyrights, his patients, retaining fees. His occupation of the Chair of Medicine had encouraged so many new students to Pavia that the university had once more become prosperous. Cardano's salary had been raised to six hundred gold crowns a year and was paid punctually. In short, his material success was all that any man could feel himself entitled to; his professional reputation in all the fields he had explored was challengeable only by the highest; his spiritual affairs were so far as we know in order. From the materials of a troubled life he had wrought an enduring edifice. It now remained to be seen how easily that edifice could be brought down.

Of those who attacked, Chiara was the first to deal an effective blow. Her promiscuous life had brought her, apart from the lascivious pleasures of her mania, nothing but the dreadful manifestations of syphilis and the barrenness caused by aborting the child of her incestuous union with Giovanni. Even after her marriage to Bartolomeo Sacco she remained unconcerned about both. Bartolomeo, however, could hardly be expected to be indifferent. "Not only have you shed upon me the great pox in the person of your unclean daughter", he wrote to Cardano; "but you have given me a wife whose demands night and day are more than can be met by the staunchest lover of couch pleasures. And when I reprimand her for her insatiable lusts she will as soon raise her dress to a servant, or would if they were not gradually learning to leave my service rather than risk the running pox. And for all this she is like a dead twig and bears nothing but her pudendum. I am to see the Cardinal about annulment, and you, bold father-in-law, about recompense for this worthless baggage". Lighthearted and punning though that letter may seem, it was not meant to be treated lightheartedly. Bartolomeo's lineage was ancient and noble; and though his escutcheon was far from spotless, there were degrees of depravity that were acceptable and those that were not. For most of the years 1557 and 1558 there were legal and ecclesiastical battles over Chiara's marriage that had the unfortunate effect of putting Cardano in a most unfavourable public light. The details have been obscured by time; but Cardano recalls the increasing distress to which he was subjected by lawyers and priests and the increasing madness of his daughter. "A young woman still, she was brought to book of the Spanish disease and her own sad flux. And I was brought to book of calumny that took me into the lawyers' maze where my father shed his years in argument. All this brought my reputation to that of an odious man; and when the time came it was remembered and weighted against me as evidence".[1]

Bartolomeo was freed of Chiara on the grounds that she was already outside the privilege of being given as a bride because of her mania and her known inability to bear children. To defend against such a prosecution in the ecclesiastical courts her counsel could only pass the blame for her infertility to the disease, and for the disease to her first lover. Since that was Giovanni, the incestuous crime was also revealed and that too set at Cardano's blame. Only by the secret purchase of a pardon for this monstrous sin could the full penalty of excommunication be avoided. Presumably the purchase was far from completed by a single contribution to a single dignitary, for Cardano writes "the exaction of the price was endless".[2] Blackmail was no less profitable in the church than in more openly criminal activities, given a victim who had in every sense much to lose.

His fame as a doctor and philosopher he could not lose—and indeed the years when troubles fell upon him as leaves in Vallombrosa, were also years when books continued to fall thickly from his pen. A book of precepts for children; a system of notation for the higher numbers; an explanation of astronomy for popular reading; another revision of his book on gambling; a method of embossing hieroglyphics on skin so that they could be learnt and identified by the blind; a system of shorthand; books

on spiritual meaning, meditation, and the transfiguration of the
body after death; and of course innumerable treatises on every
branch of medicine in which he had experience and many in
which he had none. The branches of his fame in fact continued
to spread like those of a great tree beneath which both scholarly
and unscholarly men waited for the fruit to fall. But also seep-

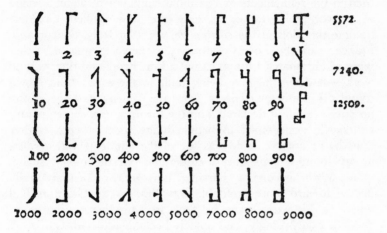

Cardano's shorthand system for writing numbers

ing through those branches was the sap of disrepute, which
people are ever ready to transform by the alchemy of rumour
and gossip into a poison.

Besides the scandal of the dissolution of Chiara's marriage
there was the infamy of Cardano's younger son Aldo to contend
with. The boy's corrupt character had at first found expression,
as Cardano had noticed, in vicious cruelties inflicted upon the
household animals. Chastised roughly by a father whose temper
had never been of the calmest and who was most greatly
incensed by such wanton persecution, the boy had directed his
viciousness elsewhere and expanded it into many additional
fields. The legal cruelties of the Inquisition suited him well, and
he made money by becoming a freelance torturer. Cardano
many times came upon accounts declaring such items as "Messer
Aldo Cardano, public executioner, for torturing by rack and
vice, Valentino Zuccaro, 3 scudi. And to the same for having in

due course burnt Zuccaro and thrown the cinders of his flesh into the river, a further 7 scudi". Such employment was, however, unpredictable. The public spectacles of the *autos-da-fé* in Portugal and Spain demanded the choicest skills in the infliction of pain. The crowds were connoisseurs of the use of the hot pincers and other contrivances of agony. Only torturers practised in the refinements by continual employment at high wages were acceptable—rather as only the most skilled toreadors become the idols of the *corrida de toros*. In Italy, Switzerland, France, and the Low Countries the spectacle was altogether more of an amateurish and casual affair. People on their way to work would see the pyre being built in the square and crowd round till master or overseer drove them away; but there were no public holidays declared, and the tortures, as a contemporary ecclesiastic accustomed to better things wrote, "were crudely done by amateurs". Aldo was one of the amateurs and needless to say found the pleasure considerable but the money inadequate. With his corrupt character, however, he not unnaturally drifted toward more profitable activities, just as Giovanni had done. In his early teens he took to gambling (perhaps not altogether surprisingly) and quickly became addicted. Cardano's interest remained throughout his life detached, a scientific study and a means of supplementing his income in harder times. But for Aldo the compulsion grew like the psychological disease it is; and like any other form of addiction it had to be fed. The money to feed it was many times stolen from Cardano's cashbox; and when that came to be more closely guarded or prove insufficient he had of course no scruples about thieving elsewhere or developing methods of cheating that many times led to violence and the dungeon. Cardano was frequently called upon to arrange his release by connivance with the authorities and the handing over of large sums of money. By 1560, when Aldo was only seventeen years old, he had become a hardened criminal upon whom, Cardano says, he had spent "thousands of crowns to release him from just punishment".[3] Only the prestige attaching to him from the scholarly world secured such favoured treatment. And that prestige diminished in inverse ratio as his notoriety as the father of infamous children increased. For the mecurial character of the Italian people is not

so inclined as that of the phlegmatic British to sympathize with
the underdog. A famous man in Britain who by grim misfortune
was the father of two indicted murderers would retain throughout his public ordeal the sympathy of the crowd. It would be
readily recognized that fame for one's achievements and notoriety for the faults of one's family are different faces of the fate
of a single individual. The warmer tempered people of southern
Europe tend to view matters differently. The house of a man's
reputation, they consider, can be kept looking innocent on the
outside while the cellars beneath collapse under the weight of
his guilt. So it was not altogether surprising that when Giovanni
in his turn attacked the edifice with wickedly severe impact
Cardano himself should come under suspicion.

In its outward appearance Giovanni's attack might almost have
been designed with personal malice toward his father as its main
weapon. In fact, though both feckless and reckless by nature, his
was too shallow a character to brood upon revenge for supposed
wrongs. In filling the office of revanchist Tartaglia was infinitely
his superior. Giovanni's malice was impulsive, the last resort of a
man in a desperate situation. And his situation in the Seroni
family had become desperate.

Since Giovanni's marriage to Brandonia and Cardano's angry
rejection of her preying family, the Seronis had adopted an attitude of persecution toward their intended benefactor. Having
proved himself profitless to them, they built around Giovanni
a corral of threat. He could not escape from it. And they
had perfected a technique of reducing and expanding its area,
so that he never quite knew how close his persecutors were or
from which direction the next shadowy fear would approach.
Since there were eight Seronis to threaten him and countless
ways of evoking terror in such a flabby character as Giovanni's,
he had little respite. They realized, of course, that they could
have despatched him to the executioner's block with the greatest
ease by handing to the authorities the evidence of his complicity
in the murder of the government official—the very threat held
over him by their original blackmail. But they were too cunning
for that. They saw equally clearly that the evidence could be far
more valuable to them if held in suspense. If they had failed in

securing the parasitic life they had planned they could at least secure something equally acceptable : a continuing supply of money. To this end Brandonia was the instrument of their strategy. She it was who laid before the cringing Giovanni the continual demands of the mother, the spinster daughters, and the hobbledehoy sons. To be forever directing his talents for evil toward the support of others was by no means Giovanni's notion of a satisfactory existence. He had foreseen no such eventuality. His evil-doing was intended to be self-supporting, not altruistic. But since it was his father who had brought about such an unpremeditated situation, he had no compunction in ensuring that his father also was its victim. With the help of Aldo, who between his spells in prison was sponging on Cardano for subsistence, he made further inroads on the father's money and treasures. Jewels, money, talismans, even books and his cherished ink-horns were from time to time stolen by the two scoundrel sons.

For some years Cardano did not relent in his rejection of Giovanni; indeed he never did relent to the extent of allowing him hearth and home. But when he heard that Brandonia, having borne a son and lost him as a consequence of the malnutrition of poverty was again a mother and destitute, he contrived through his lawyer to have the baby adopted and brought into his household. He was not stupidly sentimental enough to be unaware that the information might have been carefully sown—as indeed it was—with the very object of relieving Brandonia and Giovanni of the responsibility of unwanted children. But his compassion overcame his bitterness. "I longed for a grandson and before he was known to me as the fruit of an adulterous union between his worthless mother and an equally worthless adventurer associated with Giovanni's misspent schemes, I had decided to name him Fazio for my father and cherish him as my own. And if the knowledge of his bastardy had been mine I would have cherished him alike. For a man may be without honour and still hope to see honour spring from corruption". So wrote Cardano in *De Vita Propria*.

But little honour sprang from Giovanni's desperation. Brandonia's endless importunities as the tool of her family's rapacity, her sour temper and indifferent looks, her frequent adulteries and incompetent housewifery, drove him to plan her death as a temporary surcease. He was too stupid and too reckless to count the cost. A doctor, he had the means; a natural evil-doer, he lacked the moral conscience to fend off the temptation once it had entered his mind. He was in any case no stranger to murder, though in the previous case it had been committed quite heartlessly for pelf. This time, within the labyrinthine convolutions of his furtive mind he saw escape from the sinister threat continually surrounding him in the persons of eight Seronis. How he supposed that the despatch of one of them could aid him for long no-one can guess. He may possibly have thought vaguely of toppling the whole of the family by multiple murder, like skittles. At all events, taken up by the superficial ingenuity of his proposed escape from bondage, he straightaway ordered a servant to bake a cake and gave him a mixture to incorporate in it, explaining, according to the servant's later evidence, that it was "a potion to ease my lady of a pain she was troubled with".

At six o'clock on the evening of 15th February, 1560, a messenger arrived at Pavia university bearing from Milan a letter for Cardano. It was from the Rector of the College of Physicians and after a long, elaborate, and prevaricating introduction it stated quite bluntly that Cardano's daughter-in-law lay murdered by poison, that both his sons and the Seroni servant had been arrested, and that he must come at once to Milan, "That their innocence may be defended with that of the name of this learned College, lest it fall into disrepute by association". Cardano writes wryly of this plea on behalf of the College. "What fame and indulgence it had received in later years had been brought to it by me; and now, save for my immediate presence and proof of the non-committal of a crime of which I knew nothing, I would bring calumny upon it also. I could not but recall how such a simple thing as my own unwitting bastardy had earlier been a great barrier that I could not pass. But now, bastard or no, I was commanded to still the fluttering in the dovecotes of respectability. But all that was of little account against the wicked jolt my heart had received by the news of the crime. 'Can this be true' I asked myself. 'With shame already in my house from the rotting fruit of my loins, is there to be this barbarity against the house of medicine also?' I wracked myself with sobs for my fault that I had not proved worthy of better sons, that I had harboured in my house gamblers and men of light intent who had set an evil example that my children had followed. And I thought with woe of that morning when Giovanni had announced to me his marriage, when I saw with trembling fear in the palm of my right hand the semblance of a bloody dagger. Thus are the fates liberal with their warnings but mysterious with the means of interpreting them accurately. Lacking which, only the warning can be recognized and feared, and whether a man shall in consequence by his own interpretation and actions avoid what chiromancy may foretell, is impossible of solution".[5]

A charge of self-pity seems justified. Cardano really had little to reproach himself for regarding the environment he gave his children. His pleasure-loving, pleasure-seeking friends may have been unreliable and vulgar; but they can scarcely have been a contaminating influence. The environment in which his children chose their paths of disgrace was in fact very little different from his own. Chiara, it is true, could not be blamed for the infliction upon her of excessive sexuality, and the habits of abandonment common to the epoch would be unlikely to encourage control of it. But with her and her brothers practised by nature in the skills of deception, and lacking from too early an age a mother who might have discerned them, no direct fault can be laid at Cardano's door. Certainly not for showing bad example. It is more likely that he took refuge in the most obvious form of guilt and nourished it till it could be made to seem to account for everything. His character, like his mother's, had its weaknesses of instability. It had always beeen satisfying to him to count his physical ills and defects; now he could also find defects in his morality.

Whether or not his self-pity and the woeful wringing of his hands can be justified or explained is not important. His action following the hand-wringing and breast-beating is a far truer assessment of the stature of the man. Waiting only till the morning (night travelling being impossible), he hastened to Milan. His reputation had been detracted from somewhat since his return from Scotland—but only a little—by the nefarious doings

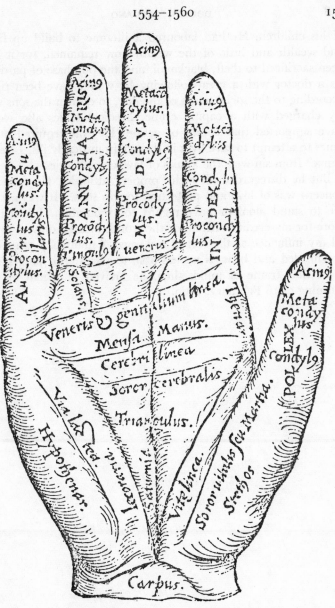

One of Cardano's chiromancy charts

of his children. He had laboured a lifetime to build up fame and wealth and little of the wealth now remained, for it had been sacrificed to theft, blackmail, and the purchase of pardons. As a doctor with a great following he would have been right, according to the social tenets of the day, to disown the sons who lay charged with a capital crime. Medical ethics also would have supported that course of action. He was required at all times to attempt to save lives in danger from fleshly ills. Lives in danger from sin were the affairs of lawyers and priests.

But he disregarded all such "proper" attitudes. His foremost concern was of love and protection for his sons. "It was not for me to stand aloof or have regard for reputation. I cared no more for my credit in Milan or the world. I cared only to throw all my influence at the feet of my sons. A man sixty years old, greyheaded and bent, is no less able to plead with judges".[6]

In that frame of mind, then, he arrived in Milan on the morning of 16 February, 1560.

17

1560

Concerned though he was to do all he could to influence favourably his sons' defence, he did not go to the prison where they lay. He was still filled with self-reproach for what he curiously thought of as his "misleading" of them and apparently could not bear to face "their accusations of my fault". It was, however, quickly known at the jail that he had arrived in the city, and Giovanni's characteristic reaction to the news was to send a message to his father asking him to stand bail for ten thousand gold crowns so that he could be released for two hours to attend a quail fight in the cathedral square. "I turned bitterly aside from the appeal. I who was not worth two thousand crowns was asked for ten that Giovanni might go to the sport. The money I had I spread instead on the tables of lawyers and independent witnesses that they might testify for Giovanni, whom I loved still".[1]

The trial was held in the great hall of the new Palazzo Marino. At the far end, beneath the banners of the Imperialist governors, was the daïs where sat the senators wearing their black robes of office and gold chains. Jurisconsults, clerks, messengers and guards were in their appointed places along the east wall. Opposite them were the witnesses. The public were contained within iron railings opposite the senators and were guarded by archers and halberdiers against making demonstrations during the prosecutors' and defenders' speeches.

According to Roman law Cardano was precluded by his relationship with the accused from offering technical evidence for the defence; but he had secured the services of five physicians from the College who, because Giovanni also was one of their fraternity, had the greatest concern to spare the name of so

august an establishment from association with a murderer. All
had made an examination of the corpse and declared unequivo-
cally that Brandonia had not died of poisoning. There were
wanting, they said, all the signs of it. Her tongue was not black,
her belly was not tumid, her hair and fingernails had not fallen
off, and there was no sign of internal corrosion. Their autopsy
was limited by the pathological knowledge of the day, and they
could in any case hardly be described as unprejudiced witnesses.
But they were listened to with great respect by the Senate, the
President, whose name was Battista Rigone, asking only one
question :

"Of what cause, then, is the woman Brandonia Cardano
lying dead?"

The witnesses conferred amongst themselves during a brief
adjournment of the trial and returned to offer the unanimous
opinion that Brandonia had died of a wasting disease called
lipyria. It was then the senators' turn to confer. They seemed
inclined to accept the doctors' opinion and to order that as there
was therefore no case to answer Giovanni should be released.
But the demands from the prosecuting counsel were too strict
for them to conclude the proceedings without hearing the cir-
cumstantial evidence regarding the administration of the poison;
and the court was adjourned again for the attackers to muster
their forces.

These were formidable. The Seroni family were masters of all
the arts of malice. They had lost by death their only link with
Giovanni, who had been a continual provider of gold, a weak-
ling who at all times could be pushed along the paths of avarice.
By their own subtleties too they had lost to Cardano's adoption
the baby that might have been used as another tool for forcing
money from Doctor Cardano. They therefore determined that
their revenge should be utterly malign. They had conspired, it
may be assumed, to give Giovanni his quietus by murder if he
should be acquitted. But it would be infinitely more satisfying to
them if legal justice worked out their malign intent for them. To
that end they had assembled every shred of evidence that would
convict him. And the prosecuting counsel now set it forth with
all possible emphasis.

The evidence of the servant to whom Giovanni had given the

mixture to put in the cake was of course of paramount importance. Nothing defending counsel could say deflected him from
his story that Giovanni had given it to him and ordered him to
incorporate it in the cake "to ease my lady of a pain she was
troubled with". Nor was he shaken in his story that he had
overheard Giovanni and Aldo plotting and that it was Aldo
who had suggested the cake as a suitable medium for the
administration of the poison. The cake had been baked and
served and Brandonia had immediately started vomiting. Was
that not irrefutable evidence, the prosecution demanded, that
the cake was poisonous? By no means, it seemed. The defending
doctors at once refuted it. Many poisons could be, and were,
taken for curative reasons. The poison of vipers was given for
elephantiasis, euphorbium for palsy, white arsenic for this very
disease, lipyria. Also, one could make a mistake and still not
intend to murder the patient, one doctor said; and the others
nodded sagely in agreement. To reinforce that argument, the
first one instanced a case in which he personally had changed
his mind at the last minute when he had been attending a child
suffering from croup, in case he had been mistaken in his prescription. "I had decided to give him a medicine called Diarob
with Turpeth to drink in little lips;* and I had already written
out the prescription and the messenger was on his way to the
pharmacist when I said to myself, 'Who knows?', I said. 'Perhaps the boy will die, that medicine being too strong an emetic,
and I shall be given the blame'. I therefore called back the
messenger, who had hardly moved four steps from the door, and
told him there was something missing which I wished to add.
Unobtrusively I tore up the first prescription and wrote another,
made up of pearls, unicorn's horn, and precious stones, that
being soothing and harmless".

The Senate listened to this and much other medical evidence.
No doubt they were confused by a science they knew nothing of
but held in respect. A present-day jury would be more demanding and less respectful and the presiding judge would see to it
that, far from being blinded by science, they had made everything clear in laymen's terms. That reasonable requirement would

* Turpeth is mercuric oxysulphate; Diarob is simply double-strength
grape juice—a kind of liquid jam vehicle for the active mercury powder.

not have obtained in 16th-century Milan; and doubtless the witnesses for the defence did all they could to add to the Senate's bewilderment by the esoteric nature of the evidence. In the event their efforts were wasted. After some days of argument during which the scribes covered sheet after sheet with the record, the members of the public scratched and fidgeted, and the senators dozed, there came the usual adjournment at the end of the afternoon. During the night, Giovanni, who according to prescribed practice had been excluded from the court during the hearing of the evidence, not only confessed to the design of the murder but added that he had "held the deed two months in contemplation" and had twice before attempted it.

That being the case, the trial was henceforth set necessarily in a new direction. His counsel was forced to adopt a plea of justification and to find advocates for mitigation of the sentence if the plea were not accepted. Though precluded by law from giving technical evidence in his son's defence, Cardano was not barred from pleading as advocate; and that he did in a speech lasting, he says, from "the hour before noon to an hour after".[1]

As we know on his own admission, Cardano was not by nature eloquent. His ways were far from being those of the conventional bedside physician. In an age notable for elaborate compliments he was often disturbingly direct. His voice was rasping and his manner frequently irascible. But on this occasion he seems to have summoned to his service both eloquence and sophistry.

His arguments were, or seem today, astonishingly casuistic. But that was the tendency of the time. Logicians did not necessarily argue in support of what they believed to be true but in support of what might be acceptable. They did not see it as absurd to argue that black is white if the opposition could be induced to believe it. Cardano did not see it as absurd to argue that Giovanni was both justified in murdering Brandonio and guiltless of the crime. He was concerned to point out that to murder by poison is scarcely to murder at all but that to murder by dagger is a capital crime. He argued also that Giovanni's confessed guilt should not lead him to the scaffold but only to exile.

The first of these arguments he explored by way of the Roman law concerning murder following provocation by faithless wives. "An act of disloyalty unblushingly confessed is greater provocation than an act detected. And Brandonia and her mother and sisters many times taunted her husband with her unfaithfulness. The child, the baby Fazio, now in my household, is not by the seed of my son but of another—as the public record office can prove. Moreover, though many wives are faithless, they respect themselves, their husbands, and their children to the extent that even though they should be killed by just wrath, they leave the reputation of their homes preserved, they do not blast the prospects of their children; but this woman cut them off from all hope. Her husband she mocked with her fornications, her first child she let die only to be rid of it—and is that not murder as great as the one her husband stands accused of? Is not therefore punishment of her faithlessness and her violence to her child justified? By our law a father is excused for the slaying of his daughter because his love can be relied upon and only a great crime by the daughter can bring his love to the anger that kills. So is it not with Giovanni? Did he not live long and patiently with her in misery, prepared to live in shame, pointed at by his neighbours as cuckolded? After such degradation, might he not himself have been killed, if not by his wife by one of his wife's paramours? Had he gone to the judges for a remedy, would not laughter have been excited, and hate among relations, and public talk and private humiliation? Was not therefore a further justification that of self-defence?"

This specious plea having been argued, Cardano cited from the legal records many examples of men who had been pardoned for slaying their detected wives, then turned to the manner of the murder. It was foolish, he said, to maintain that to kill by poison is worse than to kill by the sword or dagger. There were many authorities, he said, from Plato onward, who claimed the superior dignity and respectability of poison as an instrument of death. What man contemplating his own death would not choose the quiet poison rather than the flashing steel? "It is said of poisoning", he went on, "that it should be suppressed by additional severity because it is a crime easy to perpetrate, hard to detect. But how is that a ground for severer punishment? Martianus teaches us that small thefts by domestic servants should not be brought to trial to waste the time of the judges who have sterner matters to attend to. Yet of all offences these petty thefts are the easiest to perform. Why, then, are they not punished the most severely? Is not open contempt of law, manifested by killing by the sword, worse than the tacit respect for the law implied by the poisoner when he tries to deceive it? There is no petulance in the act of poisoning. He who kills by poison kills from some necessity. He who kills by the sword kills through anger, ambition, or licentiousness, and means to kill. He who uses poison, swaying between anger and just grief, leaves the result very much to chance. Of fifty that are poisoned, only one may die. He who drinks poison, need not drink; he who is stabbed has the knife thrust upon him, whether he will or not. If it is urged that poison is the more certain, that is baseless. It is necessary of poison that the dose be fatal, that it be all taken, and that remedies be absent or neglected. So there are for the drinker many more chances than if he were to be thrust with a dagger".

Having gone thus far in establishing that Brandonia deserved murdering—which she probably did, but that is as beside the point here as it was in the trial of her murderer—and that poisoning is a trumpery deed with little consequence and no malice behind it, to be almost welcomed by the poisoned one, Cardano now continued his casuistry by saying that although Giovanni had confessed to the crime, his confession and the deed itself were due to simple-mindedness and the wicked influence of his younger brother Aldo. (Upon receiving Giovanni's confession the court had dropped the charge against Aldo of conspiracy; so presumably Cardano felt safe in shifting some of the blame to him.) The prosecuting counsel here put, in a pointedly sneering manner, a submission that if the accused were simpleminded and incapable of understanding his own actions, so that he wantonly confessed to crimes that he had not committed, or, if he had, had done so at the instance of another whose influence he was unable to resist—if that were so, then was it not curious that such a simpleminded fellow had satisfied learned men that he had the wits to become a doctor and carry the lives of others constantly in his hands?

That, Cardano blandly assured the prosecutor, was indeed not so. "A man can be of infinite genius in the complex

demands of philosophy, medicine, the building of bridges, or a
thousand other things, and yet remain a simpleton in everyday
matters. And thus it was with this son of mine. Is it not proved
out of his own mouth? The youth acted simply. Out of his
simplicity he has confessed the whole truth, without torture,
without threats. The fact of his simplicity is most notorious. If
any of you have known him, such persons will know that I do
not lie. Ask even his accusers. If I lie upon a matter that is very
manifest, can I ask you to credit, me on doubtful points? By
simplicity he was led to take a wife without a dowry, by his
wife's relatives he was drawn into hostility against me; he has
been guilty of innumerable errors, but of no crime. His nature is
the better for his simpleness. He swears in confession as if
criminal judges would put faith in him as a wife in her husband, a parent in his child. By that you may be sure that he
tells the truth to you".

Evidently, by this time Cardano had become so ensnared by
his own sophistry that he could continue his plea with the passionate emotion of a father rather than the chosen and drily
uttered phrases of a cunning advocate. His *cri de coeur* seems to
ring through the court, perhaps creating a small stir amongst
the public in their enclosure and reaping looks of stern reproach
from the sober jurisconsults for the untimely melodrama.

"Surely my son is worthy of excuse and pardon? A youth as
simple of wit as any in the state, as I have said. Does not the
scripture plead, 'Remember not, O Lord, the sins of my youth'?
O sacred senators, how few of you have not erred gravely when
young men? Have you not all reason to be thankful, as I have,
that we have been spared the test of strength under which my
child has fallen? I thank God that my own youthful errors have
gained me only chastisement through my innocent son, and that
I am perhaps reserved for greater mercies. For Giovanni was so
simple that he had no more prudence than a boy of ten years
old, though he had a great aptitude for study. In a miserable
childhood he endured much and was the partner of all my days
of hardship. He could sometimes think and reason as well as a
man. But would you sacred senators inflict death on a lunatic
who in a lucid interval killed a man? The law inclines to
mercy; so may it not be agreed that he sinned when not in his

right mind? He is so simple that I take no more thought in the
buying of my shoes than he took in the marrying of his wife.
Was it not folly to wish to be rid of her? Could he by doing so
better his condition? Was he not foolish, if he meant murder, in
choosing as his confidants a mischievous brother and a servant
boy who would break any silence for reward? Is not his folly
emphasized by his waiting to be arrested when he was detected
instead of hastening to escape? Was not his crowning foolishness
to confess more than was suspected or any man desired to
know? And would any man in his right mind send to his father
for bail in ten thousand crowns only to seek a quail fight and
gamble on it, when his very life was at stake?"

That further wholly fallacious point established—with, perhaps, suitable pauses and gestures of appeal—Cardano turned
finally to consideration of the sentence. He did not, he said, ask
for pardon on Giovanni's behalf. That in itself seemed odd, for
the tenor of his whole speech seemed to be a plea for pardon
and nothing else. However, advancing the justification for a
reduction of the sentence, he dwelt upon the claim to consideration established by the social rank of the accused. "Is he not a
baccalaureat, a man honoured by Academy and College, a
youth noble by ancestry? He is a learned man in his profession.
Is the head matured and educated by so many nights of toil to
be cut off like the head of a man as ignorant of yesterday as of
tomorrow? Is his noble ancestry of no account? For I assure
you, masters, that no artificer or person of ignoble rank is to be
found among our forefathers".[3]

With that Cardano ended his argument; but not quite his
plea. He had, he recalls, meditated for many days on how his
final words should be phrased, and decided that they should be
simple yet powerful. "Many times I had seen the sanguine upon
the grim executioner's block and shuddered. And had I not also
seen and smelt the dreadful hulks of ships where the wretched
slaves toiled under the lash? To one of these punishments, as a
guilty murderer, my son could be sentenced. It behoved me well
to plead strongly if simply. And when it came to the doing tears
ran down my face, so that I do not feel that I failed in my
attempt".

His plea certainly was simple. "O sacred senators", he said:

"you cannot condemn a son to the galleys without condemning to a worse fate the father, who is innocent; and to kill him would be a fate worse than death to me. I beseech you, therefore, that if you prove him guilty you sentence him to perpetual exile, and spare him his life and dignity. For in that way you will also spare mine".

He then bowed to the senate and jurisconsults, stepped down from the rostrum, and returned home at once, being unable to bear the waiting in court while the verdict was being considered. "My heart was shocked by the recollection of my son's grief; I was alarmed by the impending peril; wearied by the past course of events; anxious for the future. But the speech was delivered, the struggle for the life of my first-born son was at an end. I could do no more".

It was now the fifty-third day of the trial—"And the blood-red image of the dagger in my palm glowed as if with blood and fire. I lay on my bed looking at it and calling the attention of my servant to it until at last the sentence was brought by a messenger. I had hoped for the friendly intervention of the Governor, or those members of the senate who were patients of mine and had perhaps reason for gratitude to me. But no man stretched out a hand to rescue me from an old age of sorrow. Giovanni was condemned to death. This much mercy was shown : that if peace could be made with the complainants, then his life would be spared. But no terms could be made. Giovanni had foolishly bragged to the Seroni family that my fortunes were unlimited; and they demanded, as the price of their relenting, more gold and treasure than could be found in the coffers of a king—sums that were in no way possible to raise, and I believe they knew it and were but mocking me by their demands. So all was lost".[4]

The mysterious sign of the dagger, which he had seen, or imagined, in the lines of his hand, had by the next morning vanished. During the night Giovanni had been executed in his prison. He was twenty-six years old.

18

1560-1576

From that moment, for more than ten years, Cardano's mind is weakened by sorrow and self-reproach. He is afflicted with insomnia, with "lights in the head", with an increasing concern with flagellation. The boy William is called upon to perform this service so often that he turns in disgust from his master. Now twenty years old, he finds the frequent occasions when Cardano drools and cries with impotent lusts not at all to his developing tastes. Cardano bids him go, not in anger but in the affection of a lucid moment. He arranges for the youth to be apprenticed to a tailor. Alone, he croons to his adopted grandson Fazio, lavishes every care he can afford upon the child, is often found, by patients who come to him for treatment, holding the baby in his arms and unwilling to be distracted. After a while the phase of monomania turns in another direction : he becomes a paranoiac. Shadows taunt him at every street corner, every single act of ordinary social intercourse assumes sinister stature, he hears mocking laughter in an empty house, the music of harps becomes the clash of threatening daggers, every cup of wine is poisoned by an enemy hand. These lunacies were but extensions of the guilt with which he had for long inflicted himself. He believed himself deserving of persecution for his supposed unworthiness in proving so poor an examplar to his children.

It is not surprising that disrepute now attached itself to him very easily. His prestige had for some time been diminishing as his sons and daughter brought disgrace to his door; and a man who is given to hand-wringing and breast-beating, and crying woefully of the guilt of the father for the sins of the children, has little cause to complain when people take him at his word. Even so, his fame kept disrepute of any major order at bay up to the time of Giovanni's trial. After that, the sound of rumour grew louder. Since he protested his guilt so vehemently, might not suspicion of his complicity in the murder of Brandonia be justly attached to him? His strange behaviour did nothing to lessen it. The evil Seroni family no doubt were ready at all times to foster any adverse opinion that could be established. Fuel for the fires of infamy was added by the strange fates that overtook some of those who had been concerned in the trial. The wife of Rigone, the President of the court, died in mysterious circumstances and Rigone himself was shortly afterward forced to feign death to enable him to escape a charge of murder; one senator became sick with phthisis after the trial, another fell from a bridge and was drowned; the only son of the prosecuting counsel died of smallpox; one of the Seroni brothers was condemned to death in Sicily; a jurisconsult who had assembled the evidence against Giovanni was accused of corruption and jailed; the Governor of the prison was deprived of office and became a beggar. With such fates attending so many of those who had brought Giovanni to book, it was not surprising that Cardano should be invested with an aura of evil and the designs of a sorcerer attributed to him. A mad old man who stumbled through the streets at night escaping imaginary pursuers, laughing, threatening, railing against himself, aroused little but fear. But when after a while his reason seemed to be somewhat restored and he behaved more normally, it was evident that fear had given way to oppression. His paranoia was perhaps not such a mania as it had seemed. The slings and arrows directed at him were less those of outrageous fortune than of persecution. Machinations were contrived to deprive him of his appointments. "And this was to my ability to earn and live by my work the greatest misfortune of my life. Forasmuch as I could not with any show of decency be kept in my offices, nor could I be dismissed without some more valid excuse. I could neither continue to reside in Milan with safety, nor could I depart therefrom. As I walked about the city men looked askance at me; and whenever I might be forced to exchange words with anyone, I felt that I was a disgraced man. Thus, being conscious that my company was unacceptable, I

shunned my friends. I had no notion what I should do, or
where I should go. I cannot say whether I was more wretched
in myself than I was odious to my fellows".[1]

For two years his existence seems in fact as well as in his
mind to have been nomadic. In none of his works are there
extensive records of his comings and goings. He is sometimes in
Milan, sometimes in Pavia, sometimes in Padua. He mentions
also Bologna, and from his later move to that city it appears
that he may have been vaguely investigating the possibility of
settling there. But *De Vita Propria* is largely unrevealing—as if,
when he came to recollect, in the tranquillity of his final years,
only mumblings could be heard from his years of sorrowful
amnesia. Wherever he may have been, though, if his publisher's
imprints are correct, he wrote a great number of books. Their
quality supports the supposition that they were written during
the time when his mind was unstable. They are for the most
part of philosophical kind; and their meditations veer often
from the chosen themes. He added a chapter, *De Lucto*, to a
book set aside some years before, *De Utilitate ex adversis
Capienda*, and in it exposed much of what he felt about Giovanni's crime and death, but without the shape to the narrative
that would give it much sense. A set of essays on morality was
called *Theonoston* and feebly imitated Seneca. And he was also
inspired to write a long pseudo-poetic dialogue, *Tetim, seu de
Humanis Consiliis*, which has little rhyme and less reason. But
from the same years came a treatise on *Dialectic* illustrated by
geometrical problems and theorems, and a medical textbook,
Commentary on the Anatomy of Mundinus that remained
standard for another century. Both these technical works were
of a brilliance that proved long periods of lucid creativity
amounting almost to genius.

Also belonging to these years was the sorrow visited upon him
by the death of William. "During the summer, Daldo [the tailor
to whom William was apprenticed], who had a little farm in the
country, took the youth there and let him join in the village
games, and by degrees made him into a vine-dresser. But if at
any time it chanced that William's services were also wanted at
the tailor's shop, his master would force him to return thereto in
the evening, the farm being two miles distant, and sit sewing all

the night. Besides this the boy would go dancing with the vil-
lagers, and in the course of their merry-making he fell in love
with a girl. While I was living at Milan he was taken ill of a
fever, and came to me; but, for various reasons, I did not give
proper attention to him; first, because he himself made light of
the ailment; second, because I knew not that his sickness had
been brought on by excessive toil and exposure to the sun; and
third, because when he had been seized with a similar distemper
on two or three occasions before this, he had always got well within four or five days. Besides this I was then in trouble because of
the running away of my son Aldo with one of my servants.*
What more is there to tell? Four days after I had ordered him
to be bled, messengers came to me in the night and begged me
to go and see him, for he was apparently near his end. He was
seized with convulsions and lost his senses, but I battled with the
disease and brought him round. I was obliged to return to Pavia
to resume my teaching, and William, when he was well enough
to get up, was forced to sleep in the workshop by his master,
who had been bidden to a wedding. There he suffered so much
from cold and bad food that, when he was setting out for Pavia
to seek me, he was again taken ill. His unfeeling master caused
him to be removed to the workhouse, and there he died the
following morning from the violence of the distemper, from
agony of mind, and from the cold he had suffered. I was so
heavily stricken by mischance that it seemed to me that I had
lost another son. And by my own guilt".

The pattern of remorse now repeats itself. He is sunk into
despair again—"For my lost loved youth". Many times he
whips himself "about legs, arms, and body" to expiate what he
sees as his criminal neglect in failing to save the youth. Then the
anger dies; but the sorrow remains. He writes a tender and
moving threnody Dialogus de Morte as a consolation to himself
and a memorial to the youth, then again falls into a state of
paranoia. Rivals and enemies lurk everywhere. He spies weights
carefully balanced to fall upon his head when he enters a room,
beams sawn through so that they will collapse beneath him; he

* This is the last we hear from Cardano of Aldo's career; but other
sources are more fruitful. See Rivari, E La mente di Girdamo Cardano.
Bologna 1906.

hears plots to poison him being whispered by the choirboys at mass. It is possible that some of these plots were real. His fame had often evoked jealousy in other physicians, he had always been cantankerous, and now was foolish with lunacies or silent with sorrow. There were undoubtedly voices voting to get rid of him from the Chair of Medicine at Pavia and these were presently echoed in the more powerful college at Milan. Quite suddenly, in 1563, the senate expunged his name from the list of scholars qualified and allowed to lecture, and accused him of the grave crimes of sodomy and incest. Witnesses made depositions, affidavits found their way to the notary's office, there was cunning skill shown in offering a ready sentence instead of a trial. The sentence was of perpetual exile from the State of Milan (which included Pavia); the trial would have meant torture and prison. In the depths of his madness and despair Cardano quitted Milan at the end of 1563—"Reduced once more to rags, my fortune gone, my income ceased, my rents withheld, my books impounded, my only companions prejudice and calumny".

And now at last came the moment for which Tartaglia had so long been waiting and withholding his hand. The slight humiliation he had suffered by his public defeat in the dispute with Ferrari, had been cherished and nurtured over the years; the schemes had been woven, the evidence accumulated. With Cardano at the lowest ebb of his fortunes the moment to strike was almost opportune. All the venom of Tartaglia's malevolence was released and helped to its target by circumstances so propitious to his villainy that they might have been designed expressly for its aid.

Cardano lived for seven years now in the most abject poverty. The country, wholly dominated by Spain, was exhausted by wars and burdened by heavy taxation, and the new pope, Pius V, supported the Inquisition and its cruelties to a maniacal extent. He doubtless saw the swarming forces of the Reformation ranged in ever-increasing strength. The Index was established and the Pope implemented to the uttermost degree its demands for the submission and examination of all scholarly books so that the most minute heresies might be detected in them. Scholars everywhere were fleeing the country or restricting their researches because printing was so rigidly censored. Spies of the Inquisition were everywhere. Peter Titelmann, whom Cardano had only just escaped meeting in Basel, was now pre-eminent among Inquisitorial spies and torturers, executing his infamous functions throughout Flanders, Douray, and Tournay. With fame and prestige clinging to one's name it became increasingly difficult to follow one's profession; without it, there was nothing but beggary and servitude.

Both were Cardano's lot. He was briefly in a workhouse in Padua and as briefly attached to a monastery in Gallarate, where plague had broken out and medical services were needed, however despised the man who could supply them. His wanderings are in the main untraceable except from the occasional glimpse one catches of him in the writings of contemporaries—as for example in the autobiography of De Thou, who refers to having seen "The great Cardano, now out of his wits, walking the streets shouting impieties, not dressed like any other person". He could get no employment anywhere and he put his ill-fortune down to "The treacherous times that kindled flames of want everywhere". But it was Tartaglia who was the instigator of most of the refusals that met him in College and University. It was simple enough, with the network of the Inquisition flourishing in city, vineyard, village, and public square, to keep a shadowy hand on the shoulder of any citizen, great or small. Tartaglia chose to play this cat-and-mouse game with his old enemy until 1570, accumulating great files of reports showing that Cardano was sometimes receiving a few scudi for cures he had surreptitiously effected, as in the old days in Milan when the College was determined against his entry; sometimes openly begging for alms at the gates of an academy in which he was worthy to sit in the highest seat; sometimes writing books that the censor would conveniently list in the Index; sometimes struggling against the ravages of fever, erysipelas, and gout; sometimes writing letters to his grandson Fazio, whom he had left in Milan in the care of his son-in-law Bartolomeo Sacco, but never knowing that all such letters were intercepted and never reached their destination. To ensure the continuation of all such troubles gave gleeful satisfaction to Tartaglia. But he tired of their simplicity in the end. He delayed the final blow no longer. On 13th October 1570, at Tartaglia's instance, Cardano was arrested while in Bologna. "The boy Aldo, to whom I had promised the reward of the appointment of public torturer and executioner in that city, came to me in Rome with the intelligence that his father was in Bologna awaiting an interview with the syndics. I thought to myself, 'Ah! This will be pleasant, to raise his hopes that at last the restrictions are to be lifted from him and then, an instant before the realization of those hopes, to cast him into prison. And so it was. I hastened to Bologna, and there he still sheltered, in the ruins of a hovel, awaiting an ascent to his former status. I instructed the guards to arrest him as he set out for his appointment".[2]

Tartaglia's spite by no means ended there. He allowed Cardano to languish in prison for eleven weeks without confronting him with a cause for his arrest. He was fairly looked after and was put to no torture; but that in itself added to the uncertainty, and "Uncertainty", he wrote, "is worse than knowledge when each morning comes with only a jailer for visitor, and a dumb one at that".

At last, however, he was dressed in the dreaded yellow robe of the victim of the *auto-da-fé*—"And uncertainty was mine no longer, for the grinning devils embroidered upon it are the mark of the heretic being led to the stake". But it was only another grim joke of Tartaglia's to taunt him by extending the fear of dungeon, torturer, and public burning. The uncertainty was to be prolonged still further. He was taken from the prison and set before a tribunal, where for several days he was examined regarding his opinions. It was the kind of examination likely to terrify the bravest man, for such tribunals were designed with the sole object of trapping the accused into a confession of guilt or extorting it from him by threat. And Tartaglia's patient cunning was now revealed. The members of the tribunal had before them all the evidence that had been accumulated since the days when Cardano had been offered the post of astrological adviser and physician to Pope Paul III and out of pique refused it with the unwise sarcasm that "His Holiness by his study of astrology has surely raised himself

among the greatest of such scientists and has no need of help
from such as myself". This insult now formed part of the
accusation against him. To it had been added every word that
he had ever written, or that he had spoken in the hearing of
Inquisitorial informers, which could be interpreted as heretical.
Chief among those statements and opinions was of course his
horoscope of the life of Christ, which the tribunal regarded as
an extreme blasphemy. But there were many other passages in
his works which out of context could be regarded as heretical or,
to say the least, unorthodox. He had impugned the Dominicans
in *De Varietate Rerum,* referred with approval to the wicked
tenets of Islam in *De Subtilitate,* and concerned himself with
the assumption that God is a universal spirit whose benevolence
is not restricted to holders of the Christian faith in *Paralipo-
mena.* And in his profession of doctor he had many times
ignored the papal bull forbidding "Every physician who may be
called to the bedside of a patient to visit for more than three
days unless he receives attestation that the sick man has made
fresh confession of his sins". Cardano had cared for his patients'
bodies and left their spirits to take care of themselves; and
now his neglect was formed into unanswerable accusations
against him.

The tribunal evidently found cause to mitigate the punishment of all these frightful crimes. Cardano was not subjected to
torture or death but was put back into prison with no knowledge of what fate awaited him—that perhaps being sufficient
torture in itself. There he lay for some weeks, brooding and
casting about in his mind for the name of someone near the seat
of papal authority who might influence his release. And who,
surely, but Archbishop Hamilton, who had begged to be called
upon in any circumstances in which his gratitude could be
expressed? He wrote at once, but with gloomy doubts as to the
efficacy of his plea, for had he not himself seen in the horoscope
he had cast for Hamilton and kept secret for fear it should
induce his patient to lose all hope of recovery, a dreadful and
untimely death? But he was not too late. The Archbishop sent
word by a special emissary to Rome that Cardano deserved the
benefit of any doubts that could possibly be cast upon his heretical opinions—"For he is a scholar who troubles only with

preserving and curing the bodies in which God's souls may live
to their greatest length".

Hamilton's plea was successful. It was the last help he was
called upon to render to anyone. Cardano was released in 1571.
In the same year the fate prophesied by Cardano befell Hamilton. He had governed the church in Scotland with prudence
and leniency until 1558, when he began a persecution of John
Knox's reformers which was only too well remembered when the
Reformation had become an accomplished fact. In 1563 he was
imprisoned for saying mass, but later escaped and was given
direction of the affairs of Mary, Queen of Scots. But his fate,
like hers, was already sealed. Having taken refuge in Dumbar-
ton Castle when the Queen's forces were defeated by her
enemies in 1571, he was captured and taken to Stirling to be
hanged.

For five years more after his release Cardano lived in obscurity in Rome. He ended his life there, writing the autobiographical books that reveal grief, brilliant lucidity alternating with
incomprehensible meditations and falsely remembered dates and
incidents, and longing for the companionship of his children,
whom he thought of continually. He would never have accepted
the fact, even had he known it, that Chiara had died of general
paralysis of the insane caused by syphilis, and that Aldo had
betrayed him to the Inquisition and now gleefully followed the
trade of professional torturer in the appointment given him as a
reward for his betrayal. In his last days Cardano was to be met
in the streets of Rome, walking with the strange, undirected gait
of a lunatic, curiously dressed but no longer shouting oaths and
impieties. Many of those last days were tranquil, and his last
written words were in the form of an ode in which he remembered Giovanni. He died on 20th September 1576, a man not
without greatness in an age of great and cruel men. Less than a
year later his enemy Tartaglia died also.

Reference Notes

Prologue

1 Young, M : *The Life and Times of Aonio Paleario*
2 Sadoleti, Jacobi : *Epistolae*
3 Noyes, Ella : *The Story of Milan*
4 Tasso, Bernardo : *Lettere*
5 Quoted in Young : Op. cit.
6 Bridge, J S C : *History of France from the Death of Louis XI*

Chapter One

1 Cardano, Gerolamo : *De Propria Vita*
2 Ibid
3 Cardano : *Geniturarum Exempla*
4 Peckham, John : *Perspectiva Communis* (Ed. Fazio Cardano)
5 Cardano : *De Libris Propriis*
6 Cardano : *De Propria Vita*
7 Cardano : *De Libris Propriis*
8 Ibid
9 Cardano : *De Propria Vita*
10 Peckham : Op. cit.
11 Ibid
12 Cardano : *De Propria Vita*

Chapter Two

1 Cardano : *De Libris Propriis,* the source also of the previous quotations in this chapter
2 Cardano : *De Propria Vita*
3 Ibid
4 Ibid
5 Ibid
6 Cardano : *De Libris Propriis*
7 Peckham : Op. cit.
8 Cardano : *Geniturarum Exempla*
9 Morley, Henry : *Life of Gerolamo Cardano*

Chapter Three

1 Cotterill, H B : *Italy From Dante to Tasso*
2 Ibid
3 Cardano : *De Libris Propriis*
4 Hotley, J L : *The Rise of the Dutch Republic*
5 Sarpi, Fra Paolo : *Lettere*
6 Cardano : *De Utilitate*
7 Cardano : *Liber de Ludo Aleae*
8 Cardano : *De Utilitate*

Chapter Four

1 Guicciardini, Francesco : *Storia d'Italia*
2 Gregorius, Ferdinand : *Geschichte der Stadt Rom im Mittelatter*
3 Cardano : *De Libris Propriis*
4 Ibid
5 Ibid

Chapter Five

1 This and all subsequent quotations from Cardano in this chapter are from *De Propria Vita*

Chapter Six

1 Cardano : *De Utilitate*
2 Cellini, Benvenuto : *Memoirs*
3 Cardano : *De Propria Vita*
4 Ibid
5 Ibid
6 Noyes, Ella : Opt. cit.
7 Ibid
8 Archinto, Filippo : *Lettere*
9 Bandello, G : *Novelle*

Chapter Seven

1 Cardano : *De Libris Propriis*
2 Ibid
3 Cardano : *De Sapienta*
4 Crane : Op. cit.
5 Cardano : *De Sapienta*

Chapter Eight

1 Cardano : *De Sapienta*
2 Ibid
3 Ibid
4 Ibid
5 Ibid
6 Cardano : *De Propria Vita*
7 Cardano : Preface to *De Malo Medendi Usu*
8 Ibid

Chapter Nine

1 Morley: Op. cit.
2 Cardano: *Consolatione*
3 Glussianus, Johannes (Ed): *Lettere Archinto*
4 Cardano: *De Propria Vita*
5 Ibid
6 Ibid
7 Tartaglia, Nicolo: *Memoranda*
8 Cardano: *De Propria Vita*
9 Cardano: *De Libris Propriis*
10 Ibid
11 Cardano: *Consolatione*

Chapter Ten

1 Noyes, Ella: Op. cit.
2 Cardano: *De Propria Vita*
3 Tartaglia, Nicolo: *Quesiti et Inventioni Diverse*
4 Motley, J L: Op. cit.

Chapter Twelve

1 Cardano: *Geniturarum Exemplar*
2 Ibid
3 Cardano: *Consolatione*
4 Noyes, Ella: Op. cit.
5 Cardano: *De Propria Vita*
6 Ibid
7 Laney, G: *Histoire d'Angleterre*

Chapter Thirteen

1 Cardano : *De Propria Vita*
2 Ibid
3 Morley : Op. cit., unattributed quotation
4 Dan, Père F : *Histoire de Barbarie et de ses Corsaires*
5 Cardano : *Consilia Medica*
6 Cardano : *Geniturarum Exemplar*

Chapter Fourteen

1 Cardano : *Somniorum Synesiorum*
2 Cardano : *Dialogue De Morte*
3 Ibid
4 Cardano : *Paralipomenon*

Chapter Fifteen

1 Cardano : *Consolatione*
2 Cardano : *Lettere*
3 Cardano : *Somniorum Synesiorum*
4 Cardano : *Consalatione, postscriptus*
5 Vermiglio, Peter : *Loci Communes*
6 Cardano : *De Propria Vita*
7 Cardano : *Lettere*
8 Ibid

Chapter Sixteen

1 Cardano : *De Propria Vita*
2 Ibid
3 Cardano : *Consolatione*
4 Ibid
5 Cardano : *Proxenata*
6 Ibid

Chapter Seventeen

1   Cardano : *De Propria Vita* (as are all the quotations in this chapter)

Chapter Eighteen

1   Cardano : *Paralipomenon*

Bibliography

The basic source material for this profile was the ten-volume 1663 Lyons edition of Cardano's *Opera Omnia*, and the English translation of his *Book of My Life* by Jean Stover published in New York in 1930. The other books I consulted were:

ADY, C. M. and others, *Italy, Medieval and Modern*. London 1917.
ARCHINTO, FILIPPO, *Lettere*. Basel 1603.

BANDELLO, G., *Novelle*. Florence 1577.
BEMBO, Z., *Lettere*. Florence 1584.
BERKELEY, G. F. H., *Italy in the Making*. London 1932-40.
BOULTING, William, *Tasso and his Times*. London 1907.
BRIDGE, J. S. C., *History of France From the Death of Louis XI*. London 1873.
BUONAPARTE, JACOPO, *Sacco di Roma dell' anno 1527*. Rome 1600.
BURCKHARDT, J., *The Civilization of the Renaissance in Italy*. London 1929.
BURR, C. W., *Jerome Cardan as seen by an Alienist*. Pennsylvania 1917.

CARACCIOLO, VITTORIA, *Vita di Paulo IV*. Leipsig 1803.
CELLINI, BENVENUTO, *Memoirs*. London 1843.
COTTERILL, H. B., *Italy From Dante to Tasso*. London 1919.
CRANE, T. F., *Italian Social Customs of the 16th Century*. Yale 1920.

DAN, Pére F., *Histoire de Barbarie et de ses Corsaires*. Paris 1903.

EWART, D. K., *Italy 1494-1790*. London 1909.

GIORIO, PAOLO, *La Vita di Alfonso*. Rome 1816.

GLUSSIANUS, JOHANNES (editor), *Lettere Archinto*. Milan 1903.

GUICCIARDINI, FRANCESCO, *Storia d'Italia*. Milan 1881.

HALL, V., *Life of Julius Caesar Scaliger*. New York 1903.

LANEY, G., *Histoire d'Angleterre*. Paris 1816.

MAIMONIDES, MOSES (edited by Suessman Muntner), *Treatise on Asthma*. New York 1948.

MERIMEE, PROSPER, *A Chronicle of the Reign of Charles IX.* London 1890.

MORLEY, HENRY, *Life of Gerolamo Cardano*. London 1854.

MOTLEY, J. L., *The Rise of the Dutch Republic*. London 1907.

MURATORI, F., *Antichita Estensi*. Milan 1743.

NOYES, ELLA, *The Story of Milan*. London 1908.

ORE, OYSTEIN, *Cardano the Gambling Scholar*. Princetown 1953.

PALLAVICINI, GREGORIO, *Istoria del Concilio de Trento*. Naples 1913.

RIVARI, E., *La mente di Girolamo Cardano*. Bologna 1906.

SALVATORELLI, L., *A Concise History of Italy*. London 1940.

SARPI, FRA PAOLO, *Lettere*. Basel 1603.

SEIDLITZ, W. von, *Leonardo da Vinci*. Leipsig 1903.

SHEPARD, ODELL, *The Lore of the Unicorn*. London 1930.

SADOLETI, JACOBI, *Epistolae*. Milan 1550.

SPRENGER, J. and KRAMER, H., *Malleus Maleficarum*. London 1968.

TARTAGLIA, NICOLO, *Memoranda Questi et Inventioni Diverse*. Florence 1579.

TASSO, BERNADO, *Lettere*. Bologna 1600.

TODHUNTER, I., *A History of the Mathematical Theory of Probability*. New York 1865.

TREVELYAN, G. M., *History of England*. London 1926.

VERMIGLIO, PETER, *Loci Communes*. Nuremberg 1554.

VILLARI, P., *Medieval Italy*. London 1910.

WATERS, W. G., *Jerome Cardan*. London 1898.

YOUNG, M., *The Life and Times of Aonio Paleario*. London 1860.

Index